The Making and Breaking of Affectional Bonds

'These essays, spanning 20 years of Bowlby's speaking about the forming and breaking of relationships of affection, are clear and systematic . . . They make an excellent introduction to his thought.'

British Journal of Psychiatry

'John Bowlby was a towering figure in general psychiatry, child psychiatry and psychoanalysis. More than anyone else he demonstrated the importance of real-life childhood events for the development of later psychopathology.'

The Independent

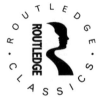

Routledge Classics contains the very best of Routledge publishing over the past century or so, books that have, by popular consent, become established as classics in their field. Drawing on a fantastic heritage of innovative writing published by Routledge and its associated imprints, this series makes available in attractive, affordable form some of the most important works of modern times.

For a complete list of titles visit
www.routledgeclassics.com

John
Bowlby

The Making and Breaking of Affectional Bonds

with a new Introduction by Richard Bowlby

 London and New York

Originally published 1979 by Tavistock Publications Limited

First published 1989 by Routledge

First published in Routledge Classics 2005
By Routledge
2 Park square, Milton Park, Abingdon, Oxon, OX14 4RN

Simultaneously published in the USA and Canada
by Routledge
270 Madison Avenue, New York, NY 10016

Reprinted 2006 (twice), 2007

Routledge is an imprint of the Taylor & Francis Group, an informa business

© 1979, 2005 R.P.L. Bowlby and others
Introduction © 2005 R.P.L. Bowlby

Typeset in Joanna by RefineCatch Limited, Bungay, Suffolk
Printed and bound in Great Britain by TJ International, Padstow, Cornwall

British Library Cataloguing in Publication Data
A catalogue record for this book is available from the British Library

Library of Congress Cataloging in Publication Data
A catalog record for this book has been requested

ISBN 10: 0–415–35481–1
ISBN 13: 978–0–415–35481–3

CONTENTS

INTRODUCTION

When my father published this collection of lectures in 1979 I had no idea it would become a classic. At the time I was a medical photographer and was about half way through his three volume 'magnum opus' *Attachment, Separation and Loss*, reading them more out of duty as a son than in a genuine thirst for knowledge. My wife and I lived next door to my parents and to get out of my child care duties I would often go round to discuss the day's events with my father and the conversation usually focused on the ideas he was writing about (and on our children) and this continued on and off for the rest of his life. The first time the full significance of his work struck me was during a family walk in the Chiltern Hills in about 1958 just after his paper on 'The nature of the child's tie to his mother' was first published. He said to me, 'You know how distressed small children get if they're lost and can't find their mother and how they keep on searching? Well, I suspect it's the same feeling that adults have when a loved one dies, they keep on searching too. I think it's the same instinct that starts in infancy and evolves throughout life as people grow up, and becomes part of adult love'. I remember thinking, well, if you're right, you're on to something really big!

My father was eager that as many people as possible should benefit from his explanations of what he had learned about making affectional bonds and the associated mental health outcomes of breaking them. However, in later life he became frustrated and rather disappointed by how reluctant people were to embrace his ideas for clinical applications. He would give some factual reasons for this, but I think he did not take account of how personally his ideas would be taken by clinicians, nor how upsetting the inferences could be. There have been many criticisms of attachment theory over the years and I believe most of these stem from the way it can press our most sensitive buttons, sometimes bringing back painful memories we would rather forget. Our sense of self is closely dependant on the few intimate attachment relationships we have or have had in our lives, especially our relationship with the person who raised us. These potent relationships, whether secure or insecure, loving or neglectful, have a profound significance for us and we need to protect our idealised perception of them vigorously; they may not be much, but they're all we've got!

Humans seem to have evolved an innate capacity to detect anything that could destabilise these vital attachment relationships, and unconscious defences seem to be activated by information about attachment theory. It's as if insight into these relationships could somehow threaten them and the clearer the information is, the more rapid and vigorous the defences that are employed; so it's hardly surprising that in the 45 years since the 'Child's tie' paper was published, attachment theory has remained unwelcomed by so many people.

By 1979 when my father had collected these seven lectures he was beginning to be more confident about the validity of his ideas and attachment theory in particular. The Strange Situation

Procedure developed by Mary Ainsworth was well established by then and producing statistically significant support for his ideas. Shortly before his death in 1990 the Adult Attachment Interview developed by Mary Main was beginning to establish itself and there were several longitudinal studies that looked very promising – which gave him great satisfaction – and these have subsequently produced unequivocal data which support his explanations and extend attachment theory into new fields.

Although my father barely mentions the role of fathers in this collection of lectures, it may not surprise readers to learn that I have a certain curiosity about his view on being a father. In his early book 'Child Care and the Growth of Love' published in 1953 by Penguin Books he writes about the role of fathers on page 15, 'In the young child's eyes father plays second fiddle and his value increases only as the child becomes more able to stand alone. . . . In what follows, therefore, while continual reference will be made to the mother-child relationship, little will be said of the father-child relationship; his value as the economic and emotional support of the mother will be assumed'[1]. This was his experience of his own father, an eminent surgeon born in 1856; a man with deeply Victorian ethics who rarely saw his six children and did not see them at all during the First World War (my father was born in 1907). However by the age of 80 my father had revised his view on the role of fathers to include accompanying children in their exploration of the world, but I'm not sure that he realised just how significant fathers would turn out to be as attachment figures for encouraging exploration and excitement.

In 2002 Karin Grossmann et al. (Social Development Vol.11, No.3, 2002) published findings from a longitudinal study in Germany called 'The Uniqueness of the Child-Father Attachment Relationship: Fathers' Sensitive and Challenging Play as a Pivotal Variable in a 16 year Longitudinal Study'. Among a wide range of other measurements, the sensitivity of fathers as exciting and challenging playmates was observed when the children were 2 years old and 6 years old. When the authors reviewed their data they found a powerful effect when mothers and fathers combined their resources. What predicted the highest social functioning young men and women in the cohort at the age of 16 and 22 years old was when mothers had provided their children with an enduring secure base, had continued to value them and had accepted their desire for exploration, and when fathers showed sensitivity to their children during exciting and challenging interactive play (not too boring nor too frightening, but appropriately exciting).

To explain the findings of 'high social functioning' for these individuals it required the authors to place equal emphasis on the child's need to play and explore with father as well as on his need to have an enduring secure base with mother. Even though these research findings have not been replicated elsewhere, one might use them to speculate that exploration, joy and excitement could be children's main motivations (as seen in their desire to return to exploration in the Strange Situation Procedure) and that the provision of a secure base is the springboard that facilitates their exploration.

If these recent findings are confirmed, they will need to be assimilated into 'attachment theory', but that could have been problematic had his theory been called 'Bowlby Theory'. My father was very careful to avoid having his name linked to it and he asked the family one supper time what he should call it. His preference was for 'attachment theory' (he no longer liked 'child's tie to his mother') and we all groaned and said why don't you call it 'love theory', but he told us that love was far more complex than this very specific biological protection mechanism that he was working on. He later explained to me that an emerging theory usually gets labelled with a person's name, but that if that happens the theory tends to become stagnant once they die. He was adamant that the theory would have to 'sink or swim on its ability to explain the observed data', and he would say 'if new and reliable data does not fit the existing theory, change the theory to take account of the new data'.

I'm sure 'The Making and Breaking of Affectional Bonds' had a profound significance for my father. When he was young he was cared for by an affectionate and playful young nanny called Minnie, but she left the family when he was about four*. He told me that he was very attached to Minnie and felt the pain of separation when their affectional bond was broken, but – although his work reminded him of this pain – he was able to work with it throughout his life. Losing a very important attachment figure and working out the importance of an enduring relationship was, I think, a large part of his motivation for a lifetime study of the affectional bond that forms between a child and his primary attachment figure.

My father was qualified as a doctor, a psychiatrist, a psychoanalyst and a psychologist. He received many prestigious honours including a CBE, honorary doctorates and fellowships including Fellow of the British Academy plus many distinguished medals and awards. But his passion was science, and the main reason he has left such an enduring legacy in the field of infant and child mental health is because his work was so deeply rooted in science, and despite the many developments and challenges to his work, this book is a lasting testimony to his success as a scientist.

RICHARD BOWLBY 2004

NOTE

1   From *Child Care and the Growth of Love* by John Bowlby, Penguin Books, 1990, p.15. Copyright © John Bowlby, 1953, 1965. Reproduced by permission of Penguin Books Ltd.

* His exact age is uncertain, it has emerged recently that he may have been nearer to six.

To my colleagues in research

Mary Salter Ainsworth
Anthony Ambrose
Mary Boston
Dorothy Heard
Christoph Heinicke
Colin Murray Parkes
James Robertson
Dina Rosenbluth
Rudolph Schaffer
Ilse Westheimer

PREFACE

From time to time during the past twenty years I have been invited to address colleagues, or a wider audience, on some formal occasion. These invitations have provided an opportunity to review research findings and to outline current thinking.

In this volume a few of these lectures, and also some contributions to symposia, have been selected for republication, in the hope that they may provide an introduction to ideas that are set out systematically and with evidence in the three volumes on *Attachment and Loss*, recently completed. Since each lecture or contribution (referred to here uniformly as lectures) was addressed to a particular audience on a particular occasion, I have thought it better to republish them in their original form rather than attempt any major revision. Each is therefore printed in a form close to that in which it was originally published, with an introductory paragraph describing the occasion and the audience. Opportunity has been taken to correct grammar and to standardize terminology and references; and a few explanatory footnotes have been added, in square brackets, where they seemed necessary. Whenever a statement calls for modification or amplification in the light of further evidence or study I have added a comment and given further references (often to chapters in one of the volumes of *Attachment and Loss*) in an annotation at the end of the lecture. A section has been omitted from Lecture 3 for reasons explained in the text.

My interest in the effects on a developing child of different forms of family experience began in 1929 when I worked for six months in what would now be called a school for maladjusted children. A decade later, after completing my psychiatric and psychoanalytic training, and working for three years in the London Child Guidance Clinic, I presented some observations in a paper entitled 'The Influence of Early Environment on the Development of Neurosis and Neurotic Character' (1940); and I was also collecting material for a monograph 'Forty-Four Juvenile Thieves' (1944, 1946). The reasons why, after the war, I selected as my special field of study the removal of a young child from home to a residential nursery or hospital rather than the broader field of parent-child interaction were several. First, it was an event that I believed could have serious ill-effects on a child's personality development. Second, there could be no debate whether it had occurred or not, in this regard contrasting strongly with the difficulty of obtaining valid information about how a parent treats a child. Third, it appeared to be a field in which preventive measures might be possible.

Whereas in this research I have endeavoured constantly to apply scientific method, I have always been keenly aware that, as in other fields of medicine, when a psychiatrist undertakes treatment or attempts prevention he must often go beyond what is acceptable scientifically. The distinction between criteria necessary in research and those acceptable in therapy and prevention is not always understood and much confusion results. In a recent lecture, 'Psychoanalysis as Art and Science' (1979), I have tried to make my position clear.

My indebtedness to the many colleagues who have worked with me over the years, and to whom this volume is dedicated, will be evident in the lectures themselves. To all of them I am deeply grateful. I am deeply grateful also to my secretary, Dorothy Southern, who has worked from the first on every one of these lectures, each in its many drafts and versions, and has done so with unfailing care and unflagging enthusiasm.

1

PSYCHOANALYSIS AND CHILD CARE*

During April and May 1956, as part of the celebrations of the centenary of Freud's birth, members of the British Psychoanalytical Society gave six public lectures in London on 'Psychoanalysis and Contemporary Thought'. I was invited to give the one on 'Psychoanalysis and Child Care'. The lectures were published two years later.

Perhaps no other field of contemporary thought shows the influence of Freud's work more clearly than that of child care. Although there had always been those who had known that the child was father to the man and that mother-love gave something indispensable to the growing infant, before Freud these

* Originally published in Sutherland, J. D. (ed.) (1958) *Psychoanalysis and Contemporary Thought*. London: Hogarth Press. Reprinted by permission of the Hogarth Press.

age-old truths had never been the subjects of scientific inquiry; they were therefore readily brushed aside as unvalidated sentimentality. Freud not only insisted on the obvious fact that the roots of our emotional life lie in infancy and early childhood, but also sought to explore in a systematic way the connection between events of early years and the structure and function of later personality.

Although, as we all know, Freud's formulations have met with much opposition – as recently as 1950 eminent psychiatrists were telling us that there was no evidence that what happens in the early years is of relevance to mental health – today many of his basic propositions are taken for granted. Not only do we find popular journals like *Picture Post** telling its public that 'the unhappy child becomes the unhappy neurotic adult' and that what is important is 'the behaviour of those amongst whom a child grows up; ... and, in the earliest years, especially the behaviour of the mother'; but these views are echoed in the publications of Whitehall. The Home Office (1955) in describing the work of its Children's Department notes that 'A child's past experiences play a vital part in his development, and continue to be important to him ...' and advises that 'The aim should be to secure as far as possible that each baby is cared for regularly by the same person'. Finally there is a report prepared by a committee appointed by the Minister of Education which deals comprehensively with all the problems of the maladjusted child (Ministry of Education 1955). It bases its recommendations uncompromisingly on such propositions as 'Modern research suggests that the most formative influences are those which the child experiences before he comes to school at all, and that certain attitudes have by then taken shape which may affect decisively the whole of his subsequent development', and 'Whether a child is happy and stable in this period (later

* [A weekly with very large circulation, subsequently discontinued.]

childhood), or unhappy and out of step with society or with his lessons, largely depends on one thing – the adequacy of his early nurture'. In celebrating the centenary of the birth of the founder of psychoanalysis it is fitting that we should record this revolution in contemporary thought.

In regard to some at least of the crucial issues of child care there is now much agreement amongst psychoanalysts and those influenced by them. All, for instance, are agreed on the vital importance of a stable and permanent relationship with a loving mother (or mother substitute) throughout infancy and childhood and of the need for awaiting maturation before venturing upon interventions such as weaning and toilet training – and, indeed, on all other steps in the child's 'education'. On other issues, however, there are differences of opinion, and in view of the relative novelty of the scientific study of these problems and their complexity, it would be surprising were there not. This is often confusing and perplexing for parents, especially those 'hot for certainty in this our life'. How much easier it would be for all of us if we knew all or at least a few more of the answers to the problem of how to bring up our children. But this is far from being the position today, and I do not for a moment wish to give the impression that it is. Yet I believe that Freud's work has provided us with some firm knowledge, and, moreover, what perhaps is even more important, shown us a fruitful way of viewing problems of child care and seeking further understanding of them.

AMBIVALENCE AND ITS REGULATION

Donald Winnicott, in his lecture on psychoanalysis and guilt,* discussed the vital role in human development of the growth of a healthy capacity for feeling guilt. He made it plain that a

* [A previous lecture in the series.]

capacity to experience guilt is a necessary attribute of the healthy person. Disagreeable though it is, like physical pain and anxiety, it is biologically indispensable and part of the price we pay for the privilege of being human beings. Further, he proceeded to describe how the capacity for feeling guilt 'implies the tolerance of ambivalence' and an acceptance of responsibility for both our love and our hate. These are themes which, largely due to the influence of Melanie Klein, have been of major interest to British analysts. It is my intention tonight to discuss further the role of ambivalence in psychic life – this inconvenient tendency we all have to get angry with and sometimes to hate the very person we most care for – and to consider those methods of child care which seem to make it easier or more difficult for a child to grow up capable of regulating this conflict in a mature and constructive way. For I believe that a principal criterion for judging the value of different methods of child care lies in the effects, beneficial or adverse, which they have on a child's developing capacity to regulate his conflict of love and hate and, through this, his capacity to experience in a healthy way his anxiety and guilt.

Let us briefly trace Freud's ideas on the theme of ambivalence. Of the countless themes running through his work, none is brighter nor more persistent than this one. It makes its first appearance in the earliest days of psychoanalysis. During his investigation of dreams Freud (1900) realized that a dream in which a loved person dies often indicates the existence of an unconscious wish that that person should die – a revelation which, if less surprising than when first advanced, is perhaps no less disturbing today than it was half a century ago. In his search for the origin of these unwelcome wishes, Freud turned to the emotional life of children and advanced what was then the bold hypothesis that in our early years it is the rule and not the exception that towards both our siblings and our parents we are impelled by feelings of anger and hatred as well as those of concern and love. Indeed, it is in this context that Freud first introduced the world to the now familiar themes of sibling rivalry and Oedipal jealousy.

In the few years after the publication of his great work on dreams, Freud's interest in infantile sexuality leads to the theme of ambivalence being less prominent in his writings. It reappears in 1909 when, in a paper on obsessional neurosis, he reminds us that 'in every neurosis we come upon the same suppressed instincts behind the symptoms . . . hatred kept suppressed in the unconscious by love. . . .' A few years later, to emphasize the key significance of this conflict, Freud (1912) introduced the term ambivalence which had recently been coined by Bleuler.

The clinical significance which Freud attached to ambivalence is reflected in his theoretical constructions. In the earlier of his two major formulations we find him postulating that intrapsychic conflict takes place between the sexual and the ego instincts. Since at the time Freud held that the aggressive impulses were a part of the ego instincts, he is able to sum up by saying that the 'sexual and ego instincts readily develop an antithesis which repeats that of love and hate' (1915). The same basic conflict is mirrored again in the second of his formulations – that concerning the conflict between life and death instincts. In this terminology we find that the ambivalence met with in neurotic patients is regarded by Freud as due either to a failure in the process of fusion of the life and death instincts or to a later breakdown of fusion – namely, defusion (1923). Once again therefore he sees the crucial clinical and theoretical problem as that of understanding how the conflict between love and hate comes to be regulated satisfactorily or not.

Opinions vary on the merits of these metapsychological formulations of Freud, and will continue to do so for many decades. Sometimes I have wondered whether the theoretical controversies they have stimulated and the abstract language in which they are couched may not have tended to blur the stark nakedness and simplicity of the conflict with which humanity is oppressed – that of getting angry with and wishing to hurt the very person who is most loved. This is a disposition of mankind which has always occupied a central position in Christian theology, and which is well known to us by such colloquial phrases as 'biting the hand that feeds us' and 'killing the goose that lays the golden eggs'. It is the theme of Oscar Wilde's *Ballad of Reading Gaol*, of which one verse runs:

> Yet each man kills the thing he loves,
>   By each let this be heard,
> Some do it with a bitter look,
>   Some with a flattering word,
> The coward does it with a kiss,
>   The brave man with a sword!

It is thanks to Freud that the significance of this conflict in man's life has been realized afresh and thanks to him, too, that it is for the first time the subject of scientific inquiry. We now know that it is the fear and guilt stemming from this conflict which underlies much psychological illness, and the inability to face this fear and guilt which underlies much character disorder, including persistent delinquency. Although our work will take a big step forward when theoretical issues are clearer, for many purposes I believe we can make good progress using such every-day concepts as love and hate, and the conflict – the inevitable conflict – which develops within us when they are directed towards one and the same person.

It will be clear then that the steps by which an infant or child progresses towards the regulation of his ambivalence are of critical import for the development of his personality. If he follows a favourable course, he will grow up not only aware of the existence within himself of contradictory impulses but able to direct and control them, and the anxiety and guilt which they engender will be bearable. If his progress is less favourable, he will be beset by impulses over which he feels he has inadequate or even no control; as a result, he will suffer acute anxiety regarding the safety of the persons he loves and be afraid, too, of the retribution which he believes will fall on his own head. This way lies danger – the danger of the personality resorting to one of a series of manoeuvres each of which creates more difficulties than it solves. For instance, fear of the punishment which is expected to result from hostile acts – and also of course from hostile intents, since it is never easy for a child to distinguish clearly one from the other – frequently leads to more aggression. Thus as often as not we find that an aggressive child is acting on the basis that attack is the best means of defence. Similarly guilt can lead to a compulsive demand for reassurance and demonstrations of love and, when these demands are not met, to further hatred and consequently further guilt. These are the vicious circles which result when the capacity to regulate love and hate develops unfavourably.

Furthermore, when a young child lacks confidence in his ability to control his threatening impulses, there is a risk that unwittingly he will turn to one or more of a multitude of primitive and rather ineffective psychic devices designed to protect his loved ones from damage and himself from the pain of a conflict that seems insoluble by other means. These psychic devices, which include repression of one or both components of the conflict – sometimes hate, sometimes love and sometimes both together – displacement, projection, over-compensation, and many others, have one thing in common: instead of the conflict being brought into the open and dealt with for what it is, all these defence mechanisms are evasions and denials that the conflict exists. Little wonder that they are so inefficient!

Before coming to our main theme – the conditions which in childhood favour or retard the development of the capacity to regulate conflict – I want to emphasize one thing more: there is nothing unhealthy about conflict. Quite the contrary: conflict is the normal state of affairs in all of us. Every day of our lives we discover afresh that if we follow one course of action we have to forgo others which are also desired; we discover, in fact, that we cannot eat our cake and have it too. Every day of our lives therefore we have the task of adjudicating between rival interests within ourselves and of regulating conflicts between irreconcilable impulses. Other animals have the same problem. Lorenz (1956) has described how formerly it was thought that only man was the victim of conflicting impulses, but how it is now known that all animals are constantly beset by impulses which are incompatible with one another, such as attack, flight, and sexual approach.

A pretty example is that of the courting robin.* Cock and then robins are dressed alike – both have red breasts. In the spring the cock robin stakes out a territory for himself and has a propensity to attack all intruders with red breasts. This means that when a potential wife enters his territory his first impulse is to attack her and her first impulse is to flee. Only when she becomes coy are the cock's hostile impulses inhibited and his courtship responses evoked. In the early phases of courtship, therefore, both sexes are in a state of conflict, the male torn between attack and sexual advance and the hen between flirtation and flight.

All recent research in psychology and biology has demonstrated unmistakably that behaviour, whether in other organisms or in man himself, is the resultant of an almost continuous conflict of interacting impulses: neither man as a species nor neurotic man as an afflicted sub-group has a monopoly of conflict. What characterizes the psychologically ill is their inability satisfactorily to regulate their conflicts.

* [Reference is to the European robin, not the American.]

CONDITIONS WHICH MAKE FOR DIFFICULTY

What, then, do we know of the conditions which make for difficulty? There can be little doubt that a principal feature of conflict which makes it difficult to regulate is the magnitude of its components. In the case of ambivalence, if either the impulse to obtain libidinal satisfaction[1] or the impulse to hurt and destroy the loved person is unusually strong, the problem of regulating the conflict will be increased. Freud realized this from the beginning. Very early in his work he dismissed the idea that it was either the existence or the nature of the conflicts experienced which distinguished the mentally healthy from those less fortunate; he suggested instead that the difference lay in that psychoneurotics exhibit 'on a magnified scale feelings of love and hatred to their parents which occur less obviously and less intensely in the minds of most children' (1900). This is a view which has been abundantly confirmed by clinical work in the past fifty years.

One key to child care is therefore so to treat a child that neither of the two impulses which endanger the loved person – libidinal greed and hatred – will become too intense. Unlike some analysts who are rather pessimistic about the innate strength of a child's impulses, I believe this condition is in most children fairly easily met provided one thing – that a child has loving parents. If a baby and young child has the love and company of his mother and soon also that of his father, he will grow up without an undue pressure of libidinal craving and without an overstrong propensity for hatred. If he does not have these things there is a likelihood that his libidinal craving will be high, which means that he will be constantly seeking love and affection, and constantly prone to hate those who fail, or seem to him to fail, to give it him.

Although the overriding need of an infant and child for love and security is now well-known, there are some who protest against it. Why should an infant make such demands? Why can't he be satisfied with less care and attention? How can we arrange things so that parents have an easier time? Perhaps one day, when we know more about a young child's libidinal needs, we may be able to describe his minimal requirements more precisely. In the meanwhile we should be wise to respect his needs and to realize that to deny them is often to generate in him powerful forces of libidinal demand and propensity to hatred which can later cause great difficulties for both him and us.

Let us not minimize the difficulties for women to which the necessity of meeting an infant's needs give rise. In days gone by, when higher education was closed to them, there was less conflict between the claims of family and career, though the frustration to able and ambitious women was none the less great. Today things are very different. We welcome women into the professions where they have come to play an indispensable part. Indeed, in all fields connected with the health and welfare of children they have been amongst our leaders. Yet this progress, like all growth and development, has brought its tensions, and many of you here tonight will know at first hand the problem of regulating the conflicting demands of family and career. The solution is not easy and it ill becomes those of us fortunate enough not to be faced with the problem to lay down the law to the other sex how they should resolve it. Let us hope that as time goes on our society, still largely organized to suit men and fathers, will adjust itself to the needs of women and mothers, and that social traditions will be evolved which will guide individuals into a wise course of action.

Let us now return to our theme and consider what happens when, for any reason, an infant's needs are not met sufficiently and at the right time. For some years now I have been interested to inquire into the ill-effects attending the separation of young children from their mothers at a time after they have formed an emotional relationship with them. There have been several reasons for my selecting this as a topic for research: first, results have immediate and valuable application; second, it is an area in which we can get comparatively firm data and so show those still hypercritical of psychoanalysis that it has good claims to scientific status; finally, the experience of a young child being separated from his mother provides us with a dramatic if tragic example of this central problem of psychopathology – the generation of conflict so great that the normal means of its regulation are shattered.

It now seems fairly certain that it is because of the intensity both of libidinal demand and of hatred which are generated that a young child's separation from his mother after he has formed an emotional relationship with her can be so damaging to the development of his personality. For some years we have known of the intense yearning and fretting which so many small children manifest on admission to hospital or residential nursery, and the desperate way in which later, after their feelings have thawed on their return home, they cling to and follow their mothers. The raised intensity of their libidinal demands needs no emphasizing. Similarly, we have learnt of the way these children reject their mothers when they first see them again and make bitter accusations against their mothers for deserting them.

Many examples of intense hostility directed against the figure most loved were recorded by Anna Freud and Dorothy Burlingham in the reports of the Hampstead Nurseries during the war. A particularly poignant example is that of Reggie who, except for an interval of two months, had spent all his life in the nurseries since he was five months old. During his stay he had formed,

> two passionate relationships to two young nurses who took care of him at different periods. The second attachment was suddenly broken at two years and eight months when his 'own' nurse married. He was completely lost and desperate after her departure, and refused to look at her when she visited him a

fortnight later. He turned his head to the other side when she spoke to him, but stared at the door, which had closed behind her, after she had left the room. In the evening in bed he sat up and said: 'My very own Mary-Ann! But I don't like her'.

(Burlingham and Freud 1944: 51.)

Experiences such as these, especially if repeated, lead to a sense of being unloved, deserted, and rejected. It is these sentiments which are expressed in the tragi-comic poems of an eleven-year-old delinquent boy whose mother had died when he was fifteen months old, and who had thenceforward experienced several substitute mothers. Here is one of the verses (whether original or not I am uncertain) which he wrote during his treatment with my colleague, Yana Popper, which seems to express what he felt to have been the reason for his having been passed from one mother-figure to another:

Jumbo had a baby dressed in green,
   wrapped it up in paper and sent it to the Queen.
The Queen did not like it because it was too fat,
She cut it up in pieces and gave it to the cat.
The cat did not like it because it was too thin,
She cut it up in pieces and gave it to the King.
The King did not like it because he was too slow,
Threw it out the window and gave it to the crow.

Later, when his therapist was going on holiday he expressed his despair of ever being loved in the words of a traditional ditty:

Oh, my little darling, I love you;
Oh, my little darling, I don't believe you do.
If you really loved me, as you say you do,
You would not go to America and leave me at the Zoo.

It is hardly surprising that such intense despair is coupled with an equally intense hatred. The more he came to care for his therapist the more prone he was to outbreaks of violent hatred, some of which came near to being dangerous. It seemed plain that the repeated separations of his early years had generated in this boy the tendency to intense ambivalence of a magnitude which his immature psychic equipment had been unable to regulate harmoniously, and that the pathological patterns of regulation adopted in his early years had persisted.

Further evidence of the way in which separation from his mother provokes in a young child both intense libidinal need and hatred is provided by a study by my colleague, Christoph Heinicke (1956). He compared the responses of two groups of children both aged between fifteen and thirty months; one group were in a residential nursery, the other in a day nursery. Though children of both groups showed a concern to regain their lost parents, those in the residential nursery expressed their desires with far more crying – in other words, more intensely; similarly, it was the children in the residential nursery and not the day nursery children who in various situations were prone to act in a violently hostile way. Though it is only an inference that this hostility is initially directed towards the absent parents, certain findings of this statistically based study are consistent with the hypothesis advanced some years ago (Bowlby 1944) that one of the major effects of mother-child separation is a great intensification of the conflict of ambivalence.

So far in considering what it is in early childhood that makes for difficulty in the regulation of ambivalence we have concentrated attention on experiences, such as maternal deprivation, which lead to libidinal craving and hatred running at specially high levels. Naturally there are many other events besides this that can give rise to trouble. Shame and fear, for instance, can make for great difficulties also. Nothing helps a child more than being able to express hostile and jealous feelings candidly, directly, and spontaneously, and there is no parental task more valuable, I believe, than being able to accept with equanimity such expressions of filial piety as 'I hate you, mummy' or 'Daddy you're a beast'. By putting up with these outbursts we show our children that we are not afraid of hatred and that we are confident it can be controlled; moreover, we provide for the child the tolerant atmosphere in which self-control can grow.

Some parents find it difficult to believe that such methods are wise or effective and feel that children should have it impressed on them that hatred and jealousy are not only bad but potentially dangerous. There are two common methods of doing this. One is by the forceful expression of disapproval by means of punishment; the other, more subtle and exploiting his guilt, is by impressing on the child his ingratitude and indicating the pain, physical and moral, which his behaviour causes his devoted parents. Although both methods are intended to control the child's evil passions, clinical experience suggests that neither are very successful and that both exact a heavy toll in unhappiness. Both methods tend to make a child afraid and guilty of his feelings, to drive them underground and so to make it more rather than less difficult for him to control them. Both tend to create difficult personalities, the first – punishment – promoting rebels and, if very severe, delinquents; the second – shame – guilty and anxiety-ridden neurotics. As in politics, so with children: in the long run tolerance of opposition pays handsome dividends.

No doubt much so far will be familiar ground: children need love, security, and tolerance. This is all very well, you may say, but are we never to frustrate our children and are we to let them do just as they please? All this avoidance of frustration, it may be said, will only lead to their growing up to be the barbarian offspring of downtrodden parents. This I believe to be a *non sequitur*; but since these conclusions are so commonly drawn it is worth dealing with them fully.

In the first place the frustrations which really matter are those concerned with a child's need for love and care from his parents. Provided these needs are met, frustrations of other kinds matter little. Not that they are particularly good for him. Indeed, one of the arts of being a good parent lies in the ability to distinguish the avoidable frustrations from the unavoidable. An immense amount of friction and anger in small children and loss of temper on the part of their parents can be avoided by such simple procedures as presenting a legitimate plaything before we intervene to remove his mother's best china, or coaxing him to bed by tactful humouring instead of demanding prompt obedience, or permitting him to select his own diet and to eat it in his own way, including, if he likes it, having a feeding bottle until he is two years of age or over. The amount of fuss and irritation which comes from expecting small children to conform to our own ideas of what, how, and when they should eat is ridiculous and tragic – the more so now that we have so many careful studies demonstrating the efficiency with which babies and young children can regulate their own diets and the convenience to ourselves when we adopt these methods (Davis 1939).

Granted, however, that there are very many nursery situations where frustration can be avoided with no inconvenience to ourselves and with beneficial effect on the tempers of all, there are others where it cannot. Fires are dangerous, china is breakable, ink stains the carpet, knives can hurt another child and also hurt the child himself. How do we avoid such catastrophes? The first rule is so to arrange the household that fires are guarded and china, ink, and knives are out of reach. The second is friendly but firm intervention. It is a curious thing how many intelligent adults think that the only alternative to letting a child run wild is to inflict punishment. A policy of firm yet friendly intervention whenever a child is doing something we wish to stop not only creates less bitterness than punishment but in the long run is far more effective. That punishment is efficient as a means of control I believe to be one of the great illusions of Western civilization. For older children and adults it has its uses as an ancillary to other methods; in the early years I believe it to be out of place both because it is unnecessary and because it can create in anxiety and hatred evils far greater than those it is intended to cure.

Fortunately with babies and young children, who are so much smaller than ourselves, friendly intervention is easy to practise; at a pinch we can pick a child up and carry him bodily away. The price it exacts is our fairly constant presence, a price which I am convinced it is wise for parents to pay. In any case, the notion that young children can be disciplined into obeying rules so that they will toe the line even in our absence is ill-founded. Young children quickly learn what we like and what we dislike, but they have not the necessary psychic apparatus always to carry out our wishes in our absence. Short of terrifying a child into inertia, the disciplining of young children is doomed to failure and those who attempt it to exhausted frustration. As an exemplar of the practice of firm but friendly intervention there is none better than the skilled nursery school teacher, and from her ways parents can learn much.

It should be noted that this technique of friendly intervention not only avoids stimulating the anger and bitterness albeit unconscious which I believe to be inseparable from punishment, but provides a child with a model for the effective regulation of his conflicts. It shows him that violence, jealousy, and greed can be curbed by peaceful means and that there is no need to resort to those drastic methods of condemnation and punishment which, when copied by a child, are apt to become distorted by his own primitive imagination into pathological guilt and ruthless self-punishment. It is, of course, a technique which is founded on the view which, following Melanie Klein, Donald Winnicott put before us – the view that there is in human beings the germ of an innate morality which, if given the opportunity to grow, provides in the child's personality the emotional foundations of moral behaviour. It is a notion which puts beside the concept of original sin, of which psychoanalysis discovers much evidence in the human heart, the concept of original concern for others or original goodness which, if given favourable circumstances, will gain the upper hand. It is a cautiously optimistic view of human nature, and one that I believe to be justified.

EMOTIONAL PROBLEMS OF PARENTS

So far we have elaborated some of the conditions of child care which seem likely to promote the healthy development of the capacity to regulate conflict. It is time to consider the problem from the parents' point of view. Are we prescribing, it may well be asked, that parents should be eternally loving, tolerant, and friendlily controlling? I think not . . . and as a parent I hope not. We parents have our angry and jealous feelings too, and whether we like it or not they are going to be expressed sometimes, if not wittingly then unwittingly. It is my belief, and certainly my hope, that if the general background of feeling and relationship is good, the occasional outburst or slap does little harm; it certainly has the advantage of relieving our own feelings, and perhaps also of demonstrating to our children that we have the same problems as they. Such spontaneous expressions of feeling, perhaps with an apology afterwards if we have gone too far, can be distinguished sharply from punishment with its formal assumption of where lie right and wrong. Bernard Shaw's dictum of never hit a child except in hot blood is a good one.

A point which those who are not parents will do well to bear in mind is that it is always far easier to care for other people's children than to care for one's own. Thanks to the emotional bond linking child to parent and parent to child, children always behave in a more babyish way with their parents than with other people. Too often one hears well-meaning people remark that a certain child behaves beautifully with them and that his babyish and difficult behaviour with his mother is due to her foolish management of him: the usual charge is that she spoils him! Such criticisms are usually misplaced and are far more often manifestations of the critic's ignorance of children than of the parent's incompetence. Inevitably the presence of mother or father evokes primitive and turbulent feelings not evoked by other people. This is true even in the bird world. Young finches quite capable of feeding themselves will at once start begging for food in an infantile way if they catch sight of their parents.

Parents then, especially mothers, are much-maligned people; maligned, I fear, particularly by professional workers, medical and non-medical alike. Even so, it would be foolish to pretend we do not make mistakes. Some mistakes are born of ignorance, but perhaps more spring from those unconscious emotional problems which stem from our own childhood. Although when examining children in a child guidance clinic it seems, in a number of cases, that the children's difficulties have arisen through the parents' ignorance of such things as the ill-effects of maternal deprivation or of premature and excessive punishment, far more frequently troubles seem to arise because parents themselves have emotional difficulties of which they are only partially aware and which they cannot control. Sometimes they have read all the latest books on child care and have been to all the lectures of psychologists in the hope that they will discover how to manage their children, but yet things have still gone wrong. Indeed, the failure of many parents with 'psychological ideas' to make a good job of their children has led cynics to decry the ideas. I believe this mistaken. What we must realize, however, is that it is not only what we do but the way that we do it which matters. Feeding on self-demand by an anxious and ambivalent mother will probably lead to far more problems than a routine regulated by the clock in the hands of one who is relaxed and happy. Similarly with modern versus old-fashioned methods of toilet training. This does not mean that modern methods are not better; it means that they are a part only of what matters and that human beings from infancy onwards are more sensitive to the emotional attitudes of those around them than to anything else.

There is nothing mysterious in this; there is no need to invoke a sixth sense. Very young children are even more alive to the significance of tones of voice, gesture, and facial expression than are adults, and from the first infants are keenly sensitive to the way they are handled.* One very anxious mother whom I am treating has told me how she has discovered that her eighteen months old boy, who she complains is intensely whiny and clinging, responds quite differently according to the way in which she leaves the room. If she jumps up and rushes out to stop the saucepan boiling over, he cries and demands that she returns. If she leaves the room quietly, he hardly notices her departure. In addition to intellectual understanding, which I do not decry, it is from a parent's sensitivity to her child's responses and from her ability to adapt intuitively to his needs that skilled child care is born.

This is nothing new. Time and again we hear it said by teachers and others that a child is suffering because of the attitude of one of his parents, usually the mother. We are told that she is overanxious or down on the child, overpossessive or rejecting, and time and again such comments are justified. But what the critics have usually failed to take into account is the unconscious origin of these unfavourable attitudes. As a result, all too often the erring parents are subjected to a mixture of exhortation and criticism, each as unhelpful and ineffective as the other.

A psychoanalytic approach at once casts a flood of light on the origin of parents' difficulties and provides a rational way

---

* See, for instance, the report by Stewart et al. (1954) on babies who cry excessively. They found this was a response to their mother's difficulties in handling them wisely.

of helping them. Very many of the difficulties encountered by parents, it will not surprise you to learn, stem from their inability to regulate their own ambivalence. When we become parents to a child powerful emotions are evoked, emotions as strong as those which bind a young child to his mother or lovers to one another. In mothers especially there is the same desire for complete possession, the same devotion, and the same withdrawal of interest from others. But, unfortunately, coupled with these delicious and loving feelings there comes all too often an admixture – I hesitate to say it – an admixture of resentment and even of hatred. The intrusion of hostility into a mother's, or a father's, feelings for the baby seems so strange and often so horrifying that some of you may find it difficult to believe. Yet it is a reality, and sometimes a grim reality, both for the parent and the child. What is its origin?

Though it is still difficult to explain this hostility, it seems plain that the feelings which are evoked in us when we become parents have a very great deal in common with the feelings that were evoked in us as children by our parents and siblings. The parent who suffered deprivation may, if she has not become incapable of feeling affection, experience an intense need to possess her child's love, and may go to great lengths to ensure that she obtains it. The parent who was jealous of a younger sibling may come to experience unreasonable hostility to the new 'little stranger' in the family, a sentiment which is particularly common in fathers. The parent whose love for his mother was shot through with antagonism for her demanding ways may come to resent and hate the demanding ways of the infant.

I believe that the trouble does not lie in the simple recurrence of old feelings – perhaps a measure of such feelings is present in every parent – but in the parent's inability to tolerate and to regulate these feelings. Those who in childhood have experienced intense ambivalence towards parents or siblings, and who have then unconsciously resorted to one of the many primitive and precarious means of resolving conflict of which I spoke earlier – repression, displacement, projection, and so on – are unprepared for the renewal of conflict when they come to be parents. Instead of recognizing the true nature of their feelings towards the child and adjusting their behaviour accordingly, they find themselves actuated by forces they know not of and are perplexed at being unable to be as loving and patient as they wish. Their difficulty is that the re-emergence of ambivalent feelings is being dealt with, without their knowledge, by the same primitive and precarious methods to which they resorted in their early childhood at a time of life when they had no better methods available. Thus the mother who is constantly apprehensive that her baby may die is unaware of the impulse in herself to kill it[2] and, adopting the same solution she adopted in childhood perhaps in regard to her death-wishes against her own mother, struggles endlessly and fruitlessly to stave off dangers from elsewhere – accidents, illnesses, the carelessness of neighbours. The father who resents the baby's monopoly of his wife and insists that her attentions are bad for it is unaware that he is motivated by the same kind of jealousy that he experienced in childhood when a younger sibling was born. The same is true of the mother impelled to possess her child's love who, by her endless self-sacrifice, tries to ensure that her child is given no excuse for any feelings other than those of love and gratitude. This mother, who at first sight appears so loving, inevitably creates great resentment in her child by her demands for his love, and equally great guilt in him through her claims to be so good a mother that no sentiment but gratitude is justified. In behaving in this way she is of course not aware that she is worthy of love, which she never had when she was small. I want to repeat that in my view it is not simply that parents are motivated in these ways which creates the difficulties for the children; what makes for trouble is the parents' ignorance of their own motives and their unwitting resort to repression, rationalization, and projection to deal with their conflicts.

There is probably nothing more damaging to a relationship than when one party attributes his own faults to the other, making him a scapegoat. Unfortunately babies and young children make perfect scapegoats since they manifest so nakedly all the sins that flesh is heir to: they are selfish, jealous, sexy, dirty, and given to tempers, obstinacy, and greed. A parent who carries a load of guilt in regard to one or other of these failings is apt to become unreasoningly intolerant of its manifestations in his child. He torments the child by his vain attempts to eradicate the vice. I recall a father who, troubled all his life by masturbation, tried to stop it in his son by putting him under a cold tap every time he found him with his hand on his genital. By acting in ways such as this the parent intensifies the child's guilt and also his fear and hatred of authority. Some of the most poisoned of parent-child relationships which lead to grave problems in the children stem from parents seeing motes in their children's eyes to avoid seeing beams in their own.

No one with an analytic orientation who has worked in a child guidance clinic can have failed to be impressed by the frequency with which these and comparable emotional problems occur in the parents of children who are referred, or the extent to which the parents' problems seem to have created or exacerbated the children's difficulties. Indeed, they are so frequent that in many clinics as much attention is given to helping the parents solve their emotional problems as to helping the children with their's. It is therefore curious to reflect that this is an aspect of psychological illness that seems to have been almost unknown to Freud and, perhaps for this reason, one to which psychoanalysts have, in my view, still to give proper attention. Yet it is one which I believe to be pregnant with hope for the future. Such limited experience as we have suggests that skilled help given to parents in the critical months before and after childbirth and in the early years of a child's life may go far in assisting them to develop the affectionate and understanding relationship to the baby that almost all of them desire. We know that an infant's earliest years when, unknown to him, the foundations of his personality are being laid are a critical period in his development. In the same way it seems that the early months and years after a baby is born are a critical period in the development of a mother and a father. In this earliest phase of parenthood parents' feelings seem more accessible than at other times, help is often both sought and welcomed and, because the relationships in the family are still plastic, it is effective. Relatively little help, if skilled and given at this time, may thus go a long way. If we are right in thinking this, then the family with a new baby is a strategic point at which to tackle the malign circle of disturbed children growing up to become disturbed parents who in turn handle their children in such a way that the next generation develops the same or similar troubles. The advantage of treating children young is now well-known; we are now advocating that parents, too, should be helped soon after they are 'born'!

The recognition that a principal cause of parental mistakes lies in the feeling that they have for their children being distorted by unconscious conflicts stemming from their own childhood is one which perhaps has not yet been absorbed into contemporary thought. Not only is it disturbing and alarming to parents, many of whom not unnaturally hope to see the family difficulty elsewhere than in their own hearts, but it is baffling to professional workers, medical and non-medical, to discover that so many of the problems that they face lie in a seemingly intangible realm, of which they have no knowledge and to help in which they have no training. None the less it is plain that this is so and, if parents are to receive the insightful help that will enable them to become the good parents they seek to be, a much greater understanding of unconscious conflict and its role in creating disturbances in the parents' management of their children will have to be achieved by professional personnel. This poses a problem of the first magnitude, and one too big for us to consider this evening.

EXTRA-PSYCHIC CONFLICT AND INTRA-PSYCHIC CONFLICT

The point of view that I am advocating, it will be seen, is based on the belief that much mental ill-health and unhappiness is due to environmental influences which it is in our power to change. In psychoanalysis as in other branches of psychiatry, indeed in all the biological sciences, the contributions respectively of nature and nurture are constantly debated. Our problem is to understand why it is that one individual grows up without great difficulties in his impulse life whilst another is beset by them. There can be no doubt that variations in hereditary endowment and in the influence of environment both play large parts. Freud himself, however, perhaps because his first environmental hypothesis (that regarding the influence of childhood seduction) proved mistaken, was cautious in implicating variations in the environment to account for the difficulties of his patients, and as he grew older seems increasingly to have believed that little could be done by environmental change to mitigate the force of infantile conflict. Many analysts have followed him in this view. Some, indeed, have not only held that those of us who are more hopeful are mistaken but have had misgivings lest by emphasizing the significance of environment we divert attention from the crucial fact of intra-psychic conflict. It must be admitted that this danger exists and that books have been written by analysts about child care which have had as their principal focus extra-psychic conflict – namely, the conflict between the child's needs and the limited opportunities provided for their satisfaction by the environment. Although, as I have already indicated, I believe this extra-psychic conflict between inner needs and external opportunity for fulfilling them to be real enough, I want to emphasize that in my view this by itself is of only limited significance for psychic development. What matters about the external environment is the extent to which the frustrations and other influences it imposes lead to the development of intra-psychic conflict of a form and intensity such that the immature psychic apparatus of the infant and young child cannot satis-factorily regulate it. It is by this criterion that we should assess the merits or demerits of child-care practices, and it is in approach-ing the problem in this way, I believe, that psychoanalysis has its principal contribution to make.

Confirmed, indeed enthusiastic, subscriber though I am to the view that the actual situations which an infant or young child experiences are of crucial significance for his development, I repeat that I do not wish to give the impression that we now know how to enable all children to grow up without emotional disturbance. Certainly I believe we already know a good deal, and that, if we were able to apply our present knowledge (and owing to the shortage of trained workers I fear this is a very big 'if'), a tremendous increase in human happiness and a tremen-dous reduction in psychological illness would follow. Neverthe-less, it would be foolish to suppose our knowledge is already such that we can guarantee that if a child has such and such experiences he will grow up without major difficulties. Not only are there such awkward problems to contend with as those aris-ing from the distorting effect of the child's fantasies and his mistaken interpretation of the world around him,[3] about which I have said nothing this evening, but there may well be difficul-ties of the origins of which at the present time we know nothing whatever. Even about those of which we have some understand-ing our knowledge is still scanty and insufficiently based on systematically collected data. The need for research is therefore great, and as our understanding increases the opportunities for fruitful research expand.

Which research approaches will prove most fruitful only the

future will reveal. All research is a gamble and we have to put our money on the horses we happen to fancy. Out of a big field my own inclination leads me to back crossbreds. It seems to me likely that studies of motivation in young children, especially the study of the way in which a mother and infant develop their highly charged relationship which is of such central concern to psychoanalysis, will gain greatly in precision and clarity from the application of concepts and research methods derived from the European school of animal behaviour studies, headed by Lorenz and Tinbergen and often known as ethology. Equally I suspect that our insight into the cognitive world that an infant and young child builds for himself, and then inhabits and finally moulds, will be greatly advanced by the concepts and research methods pioneered by Piaget. Similarly, learning theory may be expected to throw light on the learning processes which occur in the critical months and years when a new personality is born. Nevertheless, indispensable though I believe contributions of these kinds will be, they will be barren if they are not constantly interpreted in the light of knowledge gained by intimate contact with the emotional lives of children and parents in a clinical setting, using methods such as those introduced by Melanie Klein and Anna Freud and other child analysts and drawing their ultimate inspiration from the man the centenary of whose birth we celebrate this week.

NOTES

1   Here and in the paragraphs following I use traditional terminology by referring to 'libidinal demands' or 'libidinal needs'. Today I should refer instead to a child's desire for attachment or, perhaps, to a child's 'striving for a secure attachment'.

2   There are several different states of mind that can lead a mother to be constantly apprehensive lest her baby die, an unconscious wish to kill the child being only one. Amongst others are the previous loss of a child, the loss of a sibling during childhood, and the violent behaviour

of the child's father. See the discussion of phobias in Chapters 18 and 19 of *Attachment and Loss*, Volume 2.

3   I believe the distorting effects of children's fantasies have been greatly exaggerated in traditional psychoanalytic theorizing. The more details one comes to know about the events in a child's life, and about what he has been told, what he has overheard and what he has observed but is not supposed to know, the more clearly can his ideas about the world and what may happen in the future be seen as perfectly reasonable constructions. Evidence for this view is presented in the later chapters of the second volume and throughout the third volume of *Attachment and Loss*.

POSTSCRIPT

Most of the themes broached in this lecture are taken up again in later lectures in this collection. For an account of more recent work on the development of mother-infant relationships see Stern (1977).

2

AN ETHOLOGICAL APPROACH TO RESEARCH IN CHILD DEVELOPMENT*

At its annual conference in the spring of 1957 the British Psychological Society organized a symposium on 'The Contribution of Current Theories to an Understanding of Child Development'. I was invited to speak on the contribution that ethology might be expected to make, and others on associative learning theory, on psychoanalysis and on the system builders, Piaget and Freud. All four contributions were published later that year.

A central problem for both clinical and social psychology is the nature and development of a child's relationships with other people. In their approach to this problem psychologists tend to adopt one of two approaches: if they are academically and experimentally oriented they are likely to favour one or another

* Originally published in *British Journal of Medical Psychology* (1957) **30**: 230–40.

form of learning theory, if they are clinically oriented they follow one or another form of psychoanalysis. Both approaches have led to valuable work. Attempts to relate one outlook to another, however, have been few and not very successful, whilst mutual distrust and criticism between adherents have been common.

Psychoanalysts have from the first conceived of social relations in man as being mediated by instincts which stem from biological roots and impel the individual to action. Much of psychoanalytic theory has been concerned with these instincts, their serial and piecemeal emergence in ontogeny, their gradual and not always successful organization into more complex wholes, the conflicts arising when two or more are active and incompatible, the anxiety and guilt to which they give rise, the defences called into play to deal with them. Preoccupied with these primitive human passions which, because of the crude devices available to govern them, are apt as we know to our cost to carry us away to acts we later regret, psychoanalysts have often been impatient with the approach of learning theorists. In their theorizing there seems so little place for human feeling or for motivation springing from unconscious and irrational depths. To the clinician the learning theorist seems always to be struggling to cram a gallon of obstreperous human nature into a pint pot of prim theory.

Conversely learning theorists are critical of psychoanalysts. Definitions of instinct are notoriously unsatisfactory and are apt to degenerate into the allegorical. Though clinical reports are voluminous, records of systematic observation remain few. Experimental method is conspicuous by its absence. Worst of all, hypotheses are often so framed that they are not susceptible to test – a defect fatal to scientific progress. Learning theory, it is rightly contended, defines its terms, frames its hypotheses operationally, and proceeds to test them by properly designed experiments.

As one who strives to be both a clinician and a scientist I have been acutely alive to this conflict. As a clinician I have found

Freud's approach the more rewarding; not only has he drawn attention to psychological processes of immediate clinical relevance, but his series of concepts invoking a dynamic unconscious has been a practically useful way of ordering the data. Yet as a scientist I have felt uneasy about the unreliable status of many of our observations, the obscurity of many of our hypotheses and, above all, the absence of any tradition which demands that hypotheses be tested. To these defects are due I believe the controversies, too often both heated and barren, which have characterized psychoanalytic history. How, I have asked with many of my colleagues, can we subject psychoanalysis to greater scientific discipline without sacrificing its unique contributions?

It was in this frame of mind that a few years ago I came across the work of the ethologists. I was at once excited. Here was a body of biologists studying the behaviour of wild animals who were not only using concepts, such as instinct, conflict, and defence mechanism, extraordinarily like those which are used in one's day-to-day clinical work, but who made beautifully detailed descriptions of behaviour and had devised an experimental technique to subject their hypotheses to test. Today, I remain as impressed as I was then. Ethology, I believe, is studying the relevant phenomena in a scientific way. In so far as it studies the development of social behaviour, and especially the development of family relationships in lower species, I believe it to be studying behaviour analogous, and perhaps sometimes even homologous, with much of what concerns us clinically; in so far as it is using field description, hypotheses with operationally defined concepts and experiment, it is using a rigorous scientific method. True, only after it has been tried in the crucible of research endeavour shall we know whether it will prove as fruitful an approach with humans as it has with lower species. Suffice it to say that it is an approach which commends itself most warmly to me because I believe it can provide the range of concepts and data which are needed if the data and insights contributed by other approaches, notably those of psycho-analysis, learning theory and Piaget, are each to be exploited and integrated.

In reviewing briefly the main characteristics of the ethological approach let us start with the work of Darwin (1859), not only because he was an ethologist before the word had been coined, but because a basic concern of ethology is the evolution of behaviour through the process of natural selection.

In the *Origin of Species*, which was written exactly a century ago, Darwin gives a chapter to *Instinct*, in which he notes that each species is endowed with its own peculiar repertoire of behaviour patterns in the same way that it is endowed with its own peculiarities of anatomical structure. Emphasizing that 'instincts are as important as corporeal structure for the welfare of each species', he advances the hypothesis that 'all the most complex and wonderful instincts' have originated through the process of natural selection having preserved the continually accumulated variations which are biologically advantageous. He illustrates his thesis by reference to the behaviour characteristics of various species of insect, such as ants and bees, and birds, such as the cuckoo.

Since Darwin's time zoologists have been concerned to describe and catalogue those patterns of behaviour which are characteristic of a particular species and which, although in some degree variable and modifiable, are as much the hallmark of the species as the red breast of the robin or the stripes of the tiger. We cannot mistake the egg-laying activity of the female cuckoo for that of the female goose, the urination of the horse for that of the dog, the courtship of the grebes with that of the farmyard fowl. In each case the behaviour exhibited bears the stamp of the particular species and is therefore species-specific, to use a convenient if cumbersome term. Since these patterns develop in a characteristic way in almost all individuals of a species and even in individuals brought up in isolation, it is plain that they are in great measure unlearnt and inherited. On the other hand, we find individuals where they have failed to develop or in whom they have taken peculiar forms, and we may therefore conclude that the environment has an influence also. This reminds us that in living organisms neither structure nor function can develop except in an environment and that, powerful though heredity is, the precise form each takes will depend on the nature of that environment.

The species-specific behaviour patterns with which we are concerned are often amazingly complex. Consider the performance of a long-tailed tit building its beautiful lichen-covered domed nest. It comprises locating a site, collecting first moss and then spider's silk to form a platform, and gradually, by sideways movements whilst sitting on the platform, weaving the moss into a cup. The cup grows steadily as the bird weaves the nest around herself until, as a result of her continuing the process above her head, it becomes domed over. Meanwhile, lichens have been added to the outside and an entrance hole left open. Finally, the sidewalls of the entrance are strengthened and the nest lined with a profusion of soft feathers. In this astonishing performance there are fourteen distinct types of movement and combinations of movement, some common to other species, others specific to this one, each adapted to the particular environment of the nesting pair, and all so organized in time and space that the outcome is a coherent structure, unlike that met elsewhere in nature, which subserves a vital function in the survival of the race of long-tailed tits (Tinbergen, quoted by Thorpe 1956).

Other patterns are far simpler. When we shake the nest of a blackbird a number of ugly little heads bob up each with a gigantic gaping mouth; when we place a twenty-four-hour-old chick on a table with grains of food on it he will soon peck neatly and accurately at each one. But even these simpler patterns are far from simple. The gaping response of the young blackbirds is evoked and oriented by a visual gestalt as well as by shaking the nest, the pecking of the chick is so organized in space and time that each grain of food is accurately seized. Plainly such behaviour patterns cannot be simple reflexes. In the first place their organization is more complex and is directed to behaviour at a molar level; in the second it seems that once activated they often possess a motivational momentum of their own which ceases only in special circumstances.

Ethologists study these species-specific behaviour patterns, the term deriving from the Greek 'ethos' which signifies 'of the nature of the thing'.* Since Darwin's day a main purpose of this study has remained taxonomic, namely, the ordering of species with reference to their nearest relations alive and dead. For it has been found that, despite potential variability, the relative fixity of these patterns in the different species of fish and birds is such that they may be used for purposes of classification with a degree of reliability no less than that of anatomical structures. A visit to the research station of Konrad Lorenz in Germany quickly brings home Lorenz's abiding interest in revising the taxonomic classi-fication of ducks and geese by reference to their behaviour pat-terns. Similarly, a major interest of Niko Tinbergen is in making a complete descriptive inventory in terms of behaviour of the many species of gull. I emphasize this to bring home to you the extent to which these behaviour patterns are specific to the spe-cies, are inherited, and are as much of the nature of the organism as are its bones.

At this point I am aware that some of you may be a little impatient. Yes, it may be said, this is all very interesting and may be true of fish and birds, but are we sure it applies even to mammals, let alone man? Is not mammalian behaviour distinct-ive in its variability and in the part played by learning? Are we sure that in mammals there are inherited behaviour patterns?

* For discussion of terms see Tinbergen (1955).

The ethologist will answer: Yes, it is true mammalian behaviour is more variable and that learning plays a large part, but none the less each species exhibits behaviour peculiar to itself – for example, in respect of locomotion, feeding, courtship and mating, and care of young – and it seems very improbable that these patterns are wholly learnt. Furthermore, as Beach has shown for rats, and Collias and Blauvelt for goats, it is productive to study this behaviour by the same methods and to conceptualize the data in the same way as have proved so rewarding in the case of the lower vertebrates. As regards behaviour patterns there is no more sign of a sharp break between fish, birds, and mammals than as regards anatomy. On the contrary, despite the introduction of important new features, there are all the signs of an evolutionary continuum. Built-in patterns of behaviour seem to remain as important for mediating the basic biological processes of mammals as they do for other species; and in so far as Man shares the anatomical and physiological components of these processes with lower mammals, it would be odd were he not to share some at least of their behavioural components.

For taxonomic purposes the accurate description of behaviour patterns may be sufficient. For a science of behaviour, however, we need to know far more. In particular we need to know as much as possible about the nature of the conditions, both internal and external to the organism, which govern the pattern.

To our knowledge of the relevant conditions *external* to the organism, ethologists have made a major contribution. Heinroth was one of the first to point out that species-specific behaviour patterns are often activated by the perception of fairly simple visual or auditory gestalts to which they are innately sensitive. Well-known examples of this, analysed by means of experiments using dummies of various shapes and colours, are the mating response of the male stickleback, which is elicited by the perception of a shape resembling a pregnant female, the gaping response of the young herring gull, which is elicited by the perception of a red spot similar to that on the beak of an adult gull, and the attack response of the male robin which is elicited by the perception in his own territory of a bunch of red feathers similar to those on the breast of a rival male. In all three cases the response seems to be elicited by the perception of a fairly simple gestalt, known as a 'sign stimulus'.

A great deal of ethological work has been devoted to the identification of the sign stimuli which elicit the various species-specific behaviour patterns in fish and birds. In so far as many of these behaviour patterns mediate social behaviour – courtship, mating, feeding of young by parents, and following of parents by young – much light has been thrown on the nature of social interaction. In dozens of species it has been shown that behaviour subserving mating and parenthood is controlled by the perception of sign-stimuli presented by other members of the same species, such as the spread of a tail or the colour of a beak, or a song or a call, the essential characteristics of which are those of fairly simple gestalten. Such sign stimuli are known as 'social releasers'.

Whether or not the necessary external stimulus is as simple in mammals as it is in fish and birds has recently been discussed by Beach, the American psychologist, whose work on the mating behaviour of male rats and the retrieving of young by female rats is based on methods and concepts similar to those of the European and zoologically rooted school of ethology. After many experiments Beach and Jaynes (1956) have reached conclusions which at first sight appear to put rats in a different category to robins; both responses, they conclude, depend upon a stimulus pattern which is multisensory in nature. Nevertheless, they remain cautious and in a personal communication Beach has pointed out the possibility, advanced by Tinbergen, 'that if we fragmented the total maternal response of the adult female into individual sections or segments it might well turn out that each element in the sequential pattern was in fact controlled by a simple sensory cue.' Furthermore, in the same communication he has remarked that 'the behaviour of very young mammals might well be governed by simpler sensory controls than those which operate in adulthood', and that it is more than likely that certain of them are elicited by something approximating a sign stimulus. Views of this kind coming from an investigator of Beach's standing do nothing to support the view that an ethological approach is inapplicable to mammals.

Experiment may also be used to throw light on the conditions internal to the organism that are necessary for the activation of a behaviour pattern. These include maturation of body and central nervous system, as in the case of flight in growing birds, and endocrine balance, as in the case of the sexual behaviour of most if not all vertebrates. They also include whether or not the pattern has recently been activated, since it is well known that many instinctive activities are less easily evoked after they have recently been in action than after a period of quiescence. After copulation few animals are sexually aroused as easily as they were before. This and comparable changes are clearly due to a change in the state of the organism itself and in many cases experiments show that this change lies within the central nervous system. To account for these changes Lorenz (1950) postulated a series of reservoirs, each filled with 'reaction specific energy' appropriate to a particular behaviour pattern. Each reservoir was conceived as being controlled by a valve (the innate releasing mechanism or I.R.M.) which could be opened by the perception of the appropriate sign stimulus so that the reaction specific energy could be discharged in the performance of the specific behaviour. When the energy had drained away the behaviour ceased. Subsequently he supposed, the valve closed, the energy accumulated afresh and after a while the process was ready to be repeated. This psychohydraulic model of instinct with its reservoir and accumulation of 'energy' bears an obvious resemblance to the theory of instinct advanced by Freud, and it seems not improbable that both Freud and Lorenz were led to postulate similar models as the result of trying to explain similar behaviour.

However that may be, this psychohydraulic model is now discredited. It is no longer espoused either by Lorenz or Tinbergen, and for my part I hope the day will come when it is abandoned by psychoanalysts also. For it is not only mechanically crude but fails to do justice to the data. Much experimental work in recent years has demonstrated that behaviour patterns cease not because they have run out of some hypothetical energy, but because they have been 'damped down' or 'switched off'. Various psychological processes may lead to this result. One such, affecting behaviour in the long-term, is habituation. Another, affecting it in the short-term, is illustrated by experiments using oesophagostomized dogs. These have demonstrated that the acts of feeding and drinking are terminated by proprioceptive and/or interoceptive stimuli which arise in the mouth, the oesophagus, and the stomach and which in the intact animal are the outcome of the performances themselves; in other words there is a mechanism for negative feedback. Such cessation is due neither to fatigue nor to a satiation of the need for food and drink; instead the very act itself gives rise to the feedback stimuli which terminate it. (For discussion see Deutsch (1953) and Hinde (1954).)

Equally interesting are the observations of ethologists that, as well as being activated by exteroceptive stimuli, behaviour can also be terminated by them. Moynihan (1953), for instance, has demonstrated that the incubation drive of the black-headed gull is reduced only by sitting on a full clutch of properly arranged eggs. So long as this situation holds the bird sits quietly. If the eggs are removed or disarranged she becomes restless and tends to make movements of nest-building. This restlessness continues until she again experiences the stimuli arising from a full clutch properly arranged. Similarly, Hinde (1954) has observed that in early spring the mere presence of a female chaffinch leads to a reduction of the male's courtship behaviour, such as singing and searching. When she is present he is quiet, when she is absent he becomes active. In this case, where a socially relevant behaviour pattern is suppressed by sign stimuli emanating from another member of the same species, we might perhaps speak of a 'social suppressor' as a term parallel to social releaser.

It seems likely that the concepts of social releaser and social suppressor will prove valuable in the study of non-verbal social interaction in humans, and especially interaction which is emotionally toned; I refer to them again when I discuss the possible application of these ideas to child development research.

Our basic model for instinctive behaviour is thus a unit comprising a species-specific behaviour pattern governed by two complex mechanisms, one controlling its activation and the other its termination. Not infrequently it is found that a number of distinct patterns, each of which repays detailed study, are linked together in such a way that behaviour as complex as nest-building or courtship results. The biological function of these patterns and of their higher organization is to subserve the basic living processes of metabolism and reproduction; they are the counterparts at the level of molar behaviour of the physiological processes also concerned with metabolism and reproduction which have long been the subject-matter of physiology. Like the latter in each species their main forms are inherited and, as Darwin suggested a century ago, their heritable variations are as subject to natural selection as in the case of every other inherited characteristic.

Naturally this model is not unique to ethology. A similar model has been advanced independently by at least one experimental psychologist (Deutsch 1953), and much of the experimental data relating to the role of interoceptive stimuli have been collected by psychologists and physiologists. This illustrates the complementary nature of the ethological and psychological approaches. Not only are they complementary but, from William James onwards, there have been psychologists who have been keenly alive to the phenomena studied by ethologists and some, like Yerkes and Beach, have made notable contributions. The main contributions of the ethologists have been the analysis of a complex sequence of instinctive behaviour, such as courtship or nest-building, into a number of complex patterns, each governed by its own complex mechanism and together organized into a greater whole; the isolation of those features of the pattern which are inherited; and the discovery that in both their activation and their termination exteroceptive stimuli play a major part.

Before considering the application of these concepts to child development research I wish to refer briefly to two other concepts to which both ethologists and psychologists have made contributions – those of sensitive phases of development[1] and the regulation of conflict. Both concepts are central to psychoanalysis and our increasing understanding of them is of particular interest to clinicians.

In the growing individual, it has been found, species-specific behaviour patterns often go through sensitive phases of development, during which certain of their characteristics are determined either permanently or nearly so. Sensitive phases, which occur commonly though not necessarily very early in the life cycle, affect development in at least four different respects:

(a) whether or not the response develops at all,
(b) the intensity with which it is later exhibited,
(c) the precise motor form it takes,
(d) the particular stimuli that activate or terminate it.

(a) Patterns that develop in all members of a species when brought up in an 'ordinary' environment may fail altogether to appear if the environment is in some special way restricted.

Thus, it has been shown that the pecking response which is apparent in every day-old chick in an ordinary environment never develops if the chick is confined in darkness during its first fourteen days of life (Padilla 1935). Similarly, the tendency of the young mallard duckling to follow a moving object, which is at its most sensitive about sixteen hours after hatching, fails to develop if the duckling during its first forty hours has no object to follow (Weidmann 1956). In each case the sensitive period for the 'mobilization' of the response has been missed, and therefore the response fails altogether to appear.

(b) In other cases the pattern may develop in the usual way but, due to a particular experience in infancy, manifests itself in the adult with unusual intensity. A well-known example is the variation in the hoarding behaviour of adult rats after a few days of feeding frustration. Rats which as infants had been subjected at a particular age to a period of intermittent feeding frustration tended to hoard many more food pellets than rats which had not had this experience as infants. This work, of course, was carried out by an experimental psychologist, Hunt (1941).

(c) In many cases the motor part of the pattern is susceptible to learning processes and in some it has been found that this susceptibility is confined to a limited period. One of the best studied examples is the learning of song by chaffinches. Thorpe (1956) has shown that, whilst certain characteristics of the song develop even in a chaffinch brought up in isolation, others are learnt and that this learning is confined to special periods of the bird's first year. The song he learns then is the song he sings for the rest of his life.

(d) The stimuli that activate or terminate a behaviour pattern may at first be general and may later, through a process of learning, become restricted. This process of restriction, it has been found, may also be confined to a brief period of the life cycle. The famous work of Lorenz (1935) on the 'imprinting' of young goslings is well known; whereas at first a gosling will follow any moving object that is within certain wide limits of size, after a few days he will follow only the kind of objects to which he is accustomed, be it mother goose or man; and he does this irrespective of whether he has received food or comfort from the object. Another well-known example is that of the orphan lamb reared in the farmhouse who becomes fixated on humans and fails thenceforward to have social relations with sheep.

Finally, I wish to draw your attention to the discovery that in the animal's ordinary everyday life conflict situations constantly arise. The day when it was supposed that Man alone is burdened with the cross of conflicting impulses is over; now we have learned that birds and beasts of all kinds are subject to them. We have learnt, furthermore, that the outcome of such conflicts is very varied and is sometimes as maladaptive as it can be in humans. There is no necessity to confront animals with insuper-able tasks before they do silly things; a slight distraction of the mammalian mother soon after she has given birth will dislocate the sensitive mechanism regulating the potentially conflicting impulses on the one hand to eat the afterbirth and on the other to care for the young, and so lead her to continue eating so that she devours her young as well as the afterbirth. Much more I believe will be learnt from the study of the modes by which conflict is regulated in animals and the conditions which lead an individual to adopt one or another maladaptive pattern. My own expectation is that here again we shall find there are sensi-tive phases of development, the outcome of which determine what mode of regulation the individual animal henceforward habitually adopts. It is to this problem – *sensitive phases in the development of modes of regulating conflict* – that I would particularly like to see research directed; for I am confident that the solution of this problem will provide us with a key to understanding the origins of the neuroses. So far as I know no attention has yet been given to it.

APPLICATION OF ETHOLOGICAL CONCEPTS TO CHILD DEVELOPMENT RESEARCH

These then are the main concepts advanced by ethologists. Taken together they provide an approach very different to those either of learning theory or of psychoanalysis, yet by no means incompatible with substantial components of each. Whether or not the approach leads to a better understanding of the data of child development and whether or not it provides a stimulus to more and better research remains to be seen. That it provides different spectacles with which to look at things and leads to our undertaking different sorts of research seems indubitable. I will illustrate this by considering two well-known characteristics of the social behaviour of infants – their smile and their tendency from about six months onwards to attach themselves to their familiar mother-figure.

James Barrie has told us that, when the first baby smiled, the smile broke into a thousand pieces and each became a fairy. I can well believe it. Babies' smiles are powerful things, leaving mothers spellbound and enslaved. Who can doubt that the baby who most readily rewards his mother with a smile is the one who is best loved and best cared for?

In these introductory remarks I have plunged straight into an ethological description and explanation of the baby's smile. I have presented it to you as a social releaser – a behaviour pattern, probably species-specific to Man, which in ordinary circumstances matures in the early weeks of life, one of the functions of which is to evoke maternal behaviour in the mother. Further, I have suggested that it has been developed in the evolution of the human species through a differential survival rate favouring those babies who smile well. Looking at it in this way, I shall of course be concerned to identify the conditions, internal and external to the baby, that are necessary to elicit a smile and the conditions that lead to its termination. In particular I shall wonder if it is responsive to visual and auditory sign stimuli, and whether or not it is subject in any respect to sensitive phases of development. Furthermore, I shall expect to find it acting as a component in the higher organization of behaviour patterns which comprise 'attachment behaviour' in the slightly older infant – namely, the complex of behaviour uniting child to mother-figure. Work along these lines is being undertaken at the Tavistock by my colleague, Anthony Ambrose.[2]

This approach, which is readily *integrated* with learning theory, contrasts with one which is rigorously *confined* by learning theory.

About twenty years ago Dennis (1935) noted that young babies (from seven to sixteen weeks) smiled at a human face and voice. Because, as a learning theorist, he was confident that these could not be the unconditioned stimuli he undertook experiments to see if he could identify what the unconditioned stimulus was. His method was to bring up babies in such a way that as much as possible of their feeding and other care was carried out in conditions that prevented them from seeing a human face or being talked to; his expectation was that as time went on it would be possible to determine what the babies naturally smiled at. His results, however, did not confirm his expectations; the babies brought up in this way still smiled at the human face and no other stimulus condition was so effective. He noted, therefore, that he had obtained no evidence of the existence of an unconditioned stimulus for the smiling response to which the human face might have become conditioned.

None the less, Dennis could not believe his eyes. Not knowing of the work of Heinroth and Lorenz, he continued to dismiss the possibility that the human face is itself the effective unlearnt stimulus on the (mistaken) grounds that there was no evidence of a similar specificity in sensory control of unlearnt responses in animals. Instead he advanced a speculative theory that smiling comes to be aroused through a process of conditioning 'by any stimulus which announces the release of the infant from distress'. Plainly an exclusive reliance on learning theory, whilst inspiring interesting experiments, had made it difficult for him to give due weight both to his own findings and to alternative explanations.

Ten years later Spitz and Wolf (1946) published some further experimental work on the baby's smile. In a number of experiments using masks they demonstrated that in babies between two and six months of age, drawn from different racial and cultural backgrounds, the smile is evoked by the visual configurational quality of the human face. They claimed further that this configuration must include as elements two eyes in full face position and in motion. These observations have since been broadly confirmed and extended by Ahrens (1954), who also showed how the configuration necessary to evoke the smile becomes more complex with age. That at least one of the exteroceptive stimuli that evokes a smile in the two- to three-month-old infant is a fairly simple visual gestalt seems inescapable and is accepted as such by both workers. It comes as a surprise therefore to discover that, in considering the motor component of the smile, Spitz does not regard it as a built-in species-specific pattern. In personal communications he has made it plain that, instead, he regards it as a motor response which has been learnt as the result of instrumental conditioning. Likening it to the learning of language through the selection and specialized usage of naturally given phonemes, Spitz writes:

> The selection takes place by the progressive suppression (or leaving away) of the not goal-adapted patterns and by the reinforcement of the goal-adapted patterns of behaviour. This is what I mean by saying that the smiling response is an acquired behaviour pattern in response to the mother's ministration; it is there, as one of many dozens of physiognomic behaviour patterns, from the beginning; it is crystallised out of

these in response to the mother's ministrations, that is to the beginning object relations.

The notion that instead it may be built into the human baby, and by the age of six weeks or so organized all ready to be evoked by the appropriate stimuli, is not one that he readily entertains.

Yet nothing would be more likely. After all, great risks have been taken during the evolution of Man. In his equipment the balance has been tipped far in favour of flexibility of behaviour, and therefore of learning, and away from in-built fixity. Yet it would be odd were the biological security which comes from fixed patterns to have been wholly abandoned. Crying, sucking, and smiling I suspect are some of our many built-in motor patterns and represent nature's insurance against leaving everything to the hazard of learning.

Nevertheless, I recognize that the case is unproven and may never be absolutely proved. Furthermore, I want to emphasize that there is nothing in the picture I have presented that is incompatible with smiling being influenced by learning. Indeed, we have good reason to believe that it is. Recently Brackbill (1956) has reported an experiment in which two groups of babies between the ages of fourteen and eighteen weeks were subjected, for a fortnight each, to two different degrees of 'reward' for their smiles, the 'rewards' being extra attention from the experimenter. At the end of the period the two groups differed significantly in the direction expected in regard to the frequency and persistence of their smiles. The conclusion that smiling is influenced by instrumental conditioning appears from her evidence to be well based. Any further supposition that smiling is to be understood solely in terms of instrumental conditioning is not warranted by her data and, as I have already said, seems improbable. Because walking and running are improved by practice we do not conclude that they are acquired solely by learning – and if we did we should certainly be wrong!

On which way we conceptualize the baby's smile much turns; the questions on social development to which we seek answers in research will be differently framed, all our conceptions of human social interaction are likely to be different, and the clinical and educational techniques we favour will have different emphases. Let us consider briefly how it will affect research in early social development.

If we adopt the whole-hogging learning theory point of view we shall conceive of Man as an animal with no built-in social responses. We shall then be faced, as Heathers (1955) and Gewirtz (1956) have both recognized, with the problem of understanding how it happens that by the age of seven or eight months a baby has developed a strong emotionally toned tie to his mother. Much of our experimental work will then be aimed to elucidate how this development has occurred through processes of learning based on the satisfaction of physiological needs.

If on the other hand we adopt an ethological point of view, we shall proceed very differently. First, we shall be on the look-out for a number of species-specific behaviour patterns in infants that, like smiling, subserve interaction with mother. (Two that may be suspected to be of this character and that we at the Tavistock hope to study are crying and the tendency of infants to extend their arms, which seem always to be interpreted by adults as a wish to be picked up.) Having identified them, we shall attempt to analyse the releasing and suppressing stimuli to which they are sensitive. We shall expect to find that such stimuli are commonly presented by the mother and we shall look for them in such things as her appearance, the tone of her voice and the pressure of her arms. Furthermore, we shall be on the look-out for sensitive phases through which these responses may pass (both as regards their maturation and their learnt components), for a process whereby the several social responses are integrated into a more complex whole, for situations when they conflict with incompatible responses such as hostility or escape, for 'stress' situations which may lead to their temporary or possibly permanent disintegration, for their effects on maternal behaviour, and so on.

Plainly these are two very different research programmes. Apart from its squaring with conceptions stemming from psychoanalytic and other clinical experience, a main reason for preferring the ethological is that it has already proved productive in the analysis of social development and social interaction in other species, whereas learning theory, as Gewirtz himself points out, has been elaborated to account for phenomena that are relatively simpler and has therefore still to prove its relevance.

In preferring the ethological approach, I hope it is unnecessary to repeat that one is not discarding learning theory. On the contrary, for understanding many of the processes of change to which the components of instinctive patterns are subject it is indispensable and therefore complementary to ethology.

In a similar way the work of Piaget (1937) is also complementary to ethology. Even if we are right in believing that in the early months of the baby's life the releasing and suppressing stimuli of social behaviour patterns are of the nature of simple gestalts, this soon ceases to be true. Already by six months the stimuli mediating his social behaviour include complex percepts, whilst in the second year he is developing the capacity for symbolic thinking which greatly extends the stimuli that are of social significance. In understanding this change Piaget's concepts seem likely to prove indispensable. Nevertheless, we need not suppose that because an individual has become capable of utilizing more complex percepts and concepts he necessarily ceases altogether to be influenced by more primitive stimuli. On the contrary it seems not unlikely that like the chimpanzees so sympathetically described by Yerkes (1943: 35–6) we continue to be so influenced and that in conditions of anxiety and stress we are particularly sensitive to them.

This brings us to the relation of ethology to psychoanalysis. Plainly, in so far as psychoanalysis is dealing with Man as a symbol-using animal with extraordinary capacities for learning and therefore for delaying, distorting, and disguising the expression of instinctual responses, it is exploring in a region adjacent and complementary to ethology. In so far, however, as it is dealing with the instinctual responses themselves, it seems probable that the two disciplines overlap. In this context it is interesting to reflect on Freud's belief expressed over forty years ago (Freud 1915) that, for a further understanding of instinct, psychology would need to look for help from biology. As a result of developments in the biologically rooted science of ethology I believe the time has now come and that the psychoanalytic theory of instinct can be reformulated. This is not the occasion on which to attempt so large and controversial an enterprise. It will, however, be apparent that notions such as those of primary narcissism and of the control of instinct being solely the outcome of social learning will not be favoured, whereas those of primary human relationships, the inevitability of intra-psychic conflict, defences against and modes of regulating conflict, will be central. One result of such a reformulation might be a more parsimonious and consistent body of theory.

To follow up all these lines of thought by empirical research will be the task of a generation. Whether or not it is done in this country will depend on a climate of opinion in British psychology which values all these approaches, recognizes them as complementary to one another, and thus leads to undergraduates and postgraduates receiving instruction in the principles of them all.

NOTES

1   In the original version I used the then current term 'critical phase of development'. This, however, has the disadvantage of implying that

whether or not the particular development occurs is of an all or none character, which is not the case. Subsequently therefore the term 'sensitive phase of development' has been adopted to indicate that during that phase the course of development in question is no more than especially sensitive to environmental conditions.

2   See the paper by Ambrose (1963).

POSTSCRIPT

The approach advocated has been adopted with notable success by Mary Salter Ainsworth, a number of whose publications are listed in the References on pages 189–90 and also by Nicholas Blurton Jones (1972).

For an up-to-date account of ethological concepts and findings in relation to man, see Hinde (1974).

3

CHILDHOOD MOURNING AND ITS IMPLICATIONS FOR PSYCHIATRY*

Each year at its annual meeting the American Psychiatric Association invites a lecturer, usually a psychiatrist from outside the USA, to give a lecture in honour of Adolf Meyer. I was invited to give the 1961 lecture at the meeting held that spring in Chicago. It was published later in the same year.

For half a century or more there has existed a school of thought that has believed that experiences of infancy and childhood play a large part in determining whether or not an individual grows up prone to develop psychiatric illness. To the growth of this school Adolf Meyer made a great contribution. Insisting that the

* Originally published in *American Journal of Psychiatry* (1961) **118**: 481–98. Copyright, 1961, The American Psychiatric Association. Reprinted by permission.

psychiatric patient is a human being and that his disturbed thought, feeling, and behaviour must be seen in the context of the environment in which he is living and has lived, Adolf Meyer bade us pay attention to all the complex details of the patient's life history as possible clues to his illness. 'The most valuable determining feature is, as a rule, the *form of evolution* of the [symptom] complex, the time and duration and circumstances of its development'. Though I find no evidence that Adolf Meyer himself was greatly interested in experiences of earliest childhood, they lie plainly within his field of vision and are indeed a logical extension of his work.

Over the years, the belief that experiences of early childhood are of much consequence for the development of psychiatric illness has grown in strength. Nevertheless, the basic hypothesis has always been a subject of sharp controversy. Some have contended that the hypothesis is mistaken – that psychiatric illness has its roots elsewhere than in early childhood; whilst those who believe the hypothesis to be fruitful are still at sixes and sevens regarding precisely what experiences are relevant. Much of the controversy arises from the difficulty of conducting satisfactory research in this area – a difficulty deriving largely from the long gap in time between the events thought to be of consequence and the onset of the declared illness. For the science of psychopathology, therefore, the problem posed is how best to explore the area in order to reach firmer ground. My plan here is to give an account of recent developments in one line of investigation, that which has set out to understand the effect on personality development of loss of maternal care in early childhood.

During the past twenty years much evidence has accumulated pointing to a causal relationship between loss of maternal care in the early years and disturbed personality development (Bowlby 1951). Many common deviations seem to follow an experience of this kind – from delinquent character formation to a personality prone to anxiety states and depressive illness. Although there are some psychiatrists who still challenge this general conclusion, a more usual attitude is to accept that there is probably something in it and to ask for more information. A particular request has been for an hypothesis which can provide a plausible explanation of how it is that the ill-effects attributed to separation and deprivation come to follow such experiences. In what follows I shall present a sketch of where the evidence seems to be leading.

This inquiry does not follow the usual practice of psychiatric research which starts with a more or less defined clinical syndrome and then attempts to delineate the underlying pathology. Instead, it starts with a class of experience, loss of mother-figure in infancy and early childhood, and attempts thence to trace the psychological and psychopathological processes that commonly result. In physiological medicine a shift of this kind in research orientation has occurred long since. In studies, for example, of the pathology of chronic infection of the lungs, the investigator is no longer likely to start with a group of cases all showing chronic infection and attempt to discover the infective agent or agents that are at work. It is more likely he will start with a specified agent, perhaps tubercle or some newly identified virus, in order to study the physiological and physiopathological processes to which it gives rise. In so doing he may discover many things which are not immediately relevant to chronic infective pulmonary conditions. Not only may he throw light on certain acute infections and subclinical conditions, but he is almost sure to discover that infections of other organs besides lungs are the work of the pathogenic organism he has selected for study. No longer is his centre of interest a particular clinical syndrome: it is rather the manifold sequelae of a particular pathogenic agent.

The pathogenic agent with which we are concerned is loss of mother-figure during the period between about six months and six years of age. During the early months of life an infant is learning to discriminate a particular figure, usually his mother, and is developing a strong liking to be in her company. After about six months of age he shows his preferences in unmistakable fashion (Schaffer 1958). Throughout the latter half of his first year and during the whole of his second and third he is closely attached to his mother-figure, which means that he is content in her company and distressed in her absence. Even momentary separations often lead him to protest; and longer ones always do so. After the third birthday attachment behaviour is elicited a little less readily than earlier though the change is only one of degree.[1] From about his first birthday onwards other figures also, for example father or grandmother, may become important to him so that his attachment is not confined to a single figure. Nevertheless, there is usually a well-marked preference for some one person. In the light of phylogeny it is likely that the instinctual bonds that tie human young to a mother-figure are built on the same general pattern as they are in other mammalian species (Bowlby 1958; Rollman-Branch 1960; Harlow and Zimmermann 1959).

The majority of children suffer little disruption of this primary attachment in their early years of life. They live with their mother-figure and, during the relatively brief periods when she is absent, are cared for by a familiar subordinate figure. On the other hand a minority do experience disruptions. Their mother may desert or die; they may be left in hospital or institution; they may be handed from one mother-figure to another. Disruptions may be long or short, single or repeated. The experiences that belong under the general heading of maternal deprivation are thus multifarious and no one investigation can study them all. If, therefore, effective research is to be done, the experience to be studied must be fairly narrowly defined for each project.

As regards research strategies, the investigator has a choice (Ainsworth and Bowlby 1954). An obvious possibility is to examine a sample of older children and adults who had the experience in their early years with a view to discovering whether or not they differ from a comparable sample who did not have the experience. Although brilliantly adopted by Goldfarb (1955), this strategy has many practical difficulties. The principal ones are locating a suitable sample, selecting and examining appropriate controls, and finding reliable instruments to measure the features of personality that are expected to show differences. An alternative approach is to study the child's responses at the time of and in the period immediately subsequent to the experience. After spending several not very productive years following the first strategy, my research group has concentrated during most of the past decade on the second. This has been much more rewarding.

SEPARATION FROM MOTHER AND CHILDHOOD MOURNING

The basic data with which we have been concerned are observations of the behaviour of healthy children of a defined age, namely in their second and third years, exposed to a defined situation, namely a stay of limited duration in residential nursery or hospital ward in which they were cared for in traditional ways. This means that the child was removed from the care of his mother-figure and all subordinate figures and also from his familiar environment and was cared for instead in a strange place by a succession of unfamiliar people. Further data were derived from observations of his behaviour in his home during the months after his return and from reports of it from his parents. Thanks to the work of James Robertson and Christoph Heinicke we have now a considerably body of observations, some of which have been published (Robertson and Bowlby 1952; Robertson 1953a, b; Bowlby 1953; Heinicke 1956) but some of which are still to appear.[2] We feel fairly confident of the common patterns because observations by a number of other workers (Burlingham and Freud 1942, 1944; Prugh *et al.* 1953; Illingworth and Holt 1955; Roudinesco, Nicolas, and David 1952; Aubry 1955; Schaffer and Callender 1959) record substantially similar sequences of response.

In the setting described a child of from fifteen to thirty months who has had a reasonably secure relationship to his mother and has not previously been parted from her will commonly show a predictable sequence of behaviour. This can be broken into three phases according to which attitude to his mother is dominant. We have described them as phases of protest, despair, and detachment.* At first with tears and anger he demands his mother back and seems hopeful he will succeed in getting her. This is the phase of protest and may last several days. Later he becomes quieter, but to the discerning eye it is clear that as much as ever he remains preoccupied with his absent mother and still years for her return; but his hopes have faded and he is in the phase of despair. Often these two phases alternate: hope turns to despair and despair to renewed hope. Eventually, however, a greater change occurs. He seems to forget his mother so that when she comes for him he remains curiously uninterested in her, and may seem even not to recognize her. This is the third phase – that of detachment. In each of these phases the child is prone to tantrums and episodes of destructive behaviour, often of a disquietingly violent kind.

The child's behaviour on return home depends on the phase reached during the period of separation. Usually for a while he is unresponsive and undemanding; to what degree and for how long turns on the length of the separation and the frequency of visits. For example, when he has been away unvisited for a few weeks or months, and so has reached the early stages of detachment, it is likely that unresponsiveness will persist from

---

* In certain earlier papers the term 'denial' was used to denote the third phase. It has many disadvantages, however, and has been abandoned.

an hour to a day or more. When at length it breaks the intense ambivalence of his feelings for his mother is made manifest. There is a storm of feeling, intense clinging and, whenever his mother leaves him, even for a moment, acute anxiety and rage. Thence-forward, for weeks or months, his mother may be subjected to impatient demands for her presence and angry reproaches when she has been absent. When, however, he has been away for a period of more than six months or when separations have been repeated, so that he has reached an advanced stage of detachment, there is danger that he may remain permanently detached and never recover his affection for his parents.* Now in interpreting these data and in relating them to psychopathology a key concept is that of mourning. There is, indeed, good reason to believe that the sequence of responses described – protest, despair, and detachment – is a sequence that, in one variant or another, is characteristic of all forms of mourning. Following unexpected loss there seems always to be a phase of protest during which the bereaved person is striving, either in actuality or in thought and feeling, to recover the lost person[3] and is reproaching him for desertion. During this and the succeeding phase of despair, feelings are ambivalent whilst mood and action vary from an immediate expectancy expressed in an angry demand for the person's return to a despair expressed in subdued pining – or even not expressed at all. Though alternating hope and despair may continue for a long time, at length there develops some measure of emotional detachment from the person lost. After having undergone disorganization in the phase

---

* Many variables influence the child's behaviour during and after separation and this makes a brief schematic exposition difficult. The description given applies especially to the behaviour of a child who is unvisited and is cared for by nurses or others who have little insight or sympathy for his fretting. It seems likely that free visiting and more insightful care can mitigate the processes described, but there is as yet little reliable information about this.

of despair, behaviour in this phase becomes reorganized on the basis of the person's permanent absence. Though this picture of healthy mourning is not altogether familiar to psychiatrists, evidence that it is a true one seems compelling (Bowlby 1961b).

If this view is correct, the responses of young children on removal to hospital or institution must be regarded simply as variants of basic mourning processes. Irrespective of age, it seems, the same kind of responses occur and in the same sequence. Like adults, infants and young children who have lost a loved person experience grief and go through periods of mourning (Bowlby 1960b). There appear to be only two, interrelated, differences. One is that in the young the time-scale is abbreviated, though much less so than has sometimes been thought. The other, in which lies the significance for psychiatry, is that in childhood the processes leading to detachment are very apt to develop prematurely, inasmuch as they coincide with and mask strong residual yearning for, and anger with, the lost person, both of which persist, ready for expression, at an unconscious level. Because of this premature onset of detachment the mourning processes of childhood habitually[4] take a course that in older children and adults is regarded as pathological.

Once we recognize that the separation of a young child from his loved mother-figure commonly precipitates processes of mourning of a pathological sort, we are able to relate our findings to those of many other inquiries. On the one hand are the findings of workers who have taken the grief of adults as a starting-point for a study of psychopathology (Lindemann 1944; Jacobson 1957; Engel 1961). On the other are those of the more numerous investigators who have followed the traditional pattern of psychiatric research, that starts with a sick patient and tries to discern what have been the preceding events of causal significance, and who have advanced the hypothesis that loss of a loved person is in some way pathogenic.

Inquiries that have pointed to loss of a loved person as probably pathogenic are themselves of several kinds. First, there are the very numerous studies, of which Freud's *Mourning and Melancholia* (1917) is the prototype, that relate a psychiatric syndrome of relatively acute onset, such as anxiety state, depressive illness, or hysteria, to a more or less recent bereavement, and postulate that the clinical picture is to be understood as being the result of mourning having taken a pathological course. Next are the studies, almost equally numerous, that relate a psychiatric syndrome of more chronic degree, such as a tendency to episodic depression or a difficulty in experiencing feelings, to a loss that occurred in the patient's adolescence or earlier childhood. Third, there is the extensive psychoanalytic literature that seeks to relate a proneness towards psychiatric illness in later life with some failure of psychic development in early childhood. Fourth, there is a steadily accumulating series of papers that show a raised incidence of childhood bereavement in the lives of those who subsequently develop psychiatric illness; and, finally, the striking observation that individuals are apt to fall ill of psychiatric illness at an age which appears to be determined by an episode in their childhood when they suffered the loss of a parent – the so-called anniversary reactions.

Now it is certainly not possible in a single lecture to discuss systematically the relevance of the evidence derived from each of these sources. The most that can be done is to draw on a few typical studies from each field (but excluding anniversary reactions) and to indicate briefly how these findings appear to fit together. Since, however, the whole thesis turns on the nature of the processes at work in mourning and especially those present in the first phase, it is necessary to give them further attention.

URGES TO RECOVER AND TO REPROACH THE LOST PERSON: THEIR ROLE IN PSYCHOPATHOLOGY

Anger, it is not always realized, is an immediate, common, and perhaps invariable response to loss. Instead of anger indicating that mourning is running a pathological course – a view suggested by Freud and rather commonly held – evidence makes it clear that anger, including anger with the person lost, is an integral part of the grief reaction. The function of this anger appears to be to add punch to the strenuous efforts both to recover the lost person and to dissuade him or her from deserting again that are the hallmarks of the first phase of mourning. Since this phase has not only been given little attention hitherto but appears crucial for an understanding of psychopathology, it is necessary to explore it more fully.

Because in cases of death an angry effort to recover the lost person is so obviously futile there has been a tendency to regard it as itself pathological. I believe this to be mistaken. So far from being pathological, the evidence suggests that the overt expression of this powerful urge, unrealistic and hopeless though it may be, is a necessary condition for mourning to run a healthy course. Only after every effort has been made to recover the person lost, it seems, is the individual in a mood to admit defeat and to orient himself afresh to a world from which the loved person is accepted as irretrievably missing. Protest, including an angry demand for the person's return and reproach against him or her for deserting, is as much a part of an *adult's* response to loss, especially a sudden loss, as of a young child's.

This may seem puzzling. How comes it that such demands and reproaches should be made even when the person is so plainly beyond recall? Why such gross unrealism? There is I believe a good answer: it stems from evolution theory.

In the first place, a review of the behavioural responses to loss that are shown by non-human species – birds, lower mammals, and primates – suggests that these responses have ancient biological roots. Though not well recorded, such information as is available shows that many if not all the features described for humans – anxiety and protest, despair and disorganization, detachment and reorganization – are the rule also in many other species.*

In the second place, it is not difficult to see why these responses should have been evolved. In the wild to lose contact with the immediate family group is extremely dangerous, especially for the young. It is, therefore, in the interests of both individual safety and species reproduction that there should be strong bonds tying together the members of a family or of an extended family; and this requires that every separation, however brief, should be responded to by an immediate, automatic, and strong effort both to recover the family, especially the member to whom attachment is closest, and to discourage that member from going away again. For this reason, it is suggested, the inherited determinants of behaviour (often termed instinctual) have evolved in such a way that the standard responses to loss of loved persons are always urges first to recover them and then to scold them. If, however, the urges to recover and scold are automatic responses built into the organism, it follows that they will come into action in response to *any* and *every* loss and without discriminating between those that are really retrievable and those, statistically rare, that are not. It is an hypothesis of this kind, I believe, that explains why a bereaved person commonly experiences a compelling urge to recover the person even when

---

* Evidence is reviewed by Bowlby (1961b) and Pollock (1961). To give an example quoted by Pollock: a male chimpanzee who had lost his mate is recorded to have made repeated efforts to arouse her. He yelled with rage and at times expressed his anger by snatching at the short hairs of his head. Later there was crying and mourning. As time wore on he became more closely attached to his keeper and more angry than he had been hitherto when the keeper left him.

he knows the attempt to be hopeless and to reproach him or her even when he knows reproach to be irrational.

If then neither the futile effort to recover the lost person nor angry reproaches against him or her for deserting are signs of pathology, in what ways, we may ask, is pathological mourning distinguished from mourning that is healthy? Examination of the evidence suggests that one of the main characteristics of pathological mourning is an inability to express overtly these urges to recover and scold the lost person, with all the yearning for and anger with the deserter that they entail. Instead of its overt expression, which though stormy and fruitless leads on to a healthy outcome, the urges to recover and reproach with all their ambivalence of feeling have become split off and repressed. Thenceforward, they continue as active systems within the personality but, unable to find overt and direct expression, come to influence feeling and behaviour in strange and distorted ways. Hence many forms of character disturbance and neurotic illness.

Let me give a brief illustration of one such form: it is drawn from a case reported by Helene Deutsch (1937). When he came for analysis in his early thirties, this man was without apparent neurotic difficulties. The clinical picture, however, was one of a wooden and affectionless character. Helene Deutsch describes how 'he showed complete blocking of affect without the slightest insight . . . He had no love relationships, no friendships, no real interests of any sort. To all kinds of experience he showed the same dull and apathetic reaction. There was no endeavour and no disappointment . . . There were no reactions of grief at the loss of individuals near to him, no unfriendly feelings and no aggressive impulses.' How did this barren and crippled personality develop? In the light of an hypothesis regarding childhood mourning, the history together with material stemming from analysis enable us to construct a plausible account.

First, history: when he was five years old his mother had died and it was related that he had reacted to her loss without any feeling.[5] Thenceforward, moreover, he had retained no recollection of any events prior to her death. Second, material from analysis: he described how through several years of later childhood he used to leave his bedroom door open 'in the hope that a large dog would come to him, be very kind to him, and fulfil all his wishes'. Associated with this fantasy was a vivid childhood memory of a bitch which had left her puppies alone and helpless when she had died shortly after their birth. Although in this fantasy the hidden longing for his lost mother seems plainly evident, it is not expressed in a simple direct way. Instead, all memories of his mother had disappeared from consciousness and, in so far as any conscious affects towards her could be discerned, they were hostile.

To explain the course of development in this case the hypothesis I am advancing (and one that is not very different to Helene Deutsch's) is that, following his mother's death, instead of there being a full expression of his urge to recover his mother and his anger at her desertion, his mourning had moved on precipitately to a condition of detachment. In so doing the yearning and the anger had become locked inside him, potentially active but shut off from the world, and only the remainder of his personality had been left free for further development. As a result he grew up gravely impoverished. If this hypothesis is valid, the task of treatment is to help the patient to recover his latent longing for his lost mother and his latent anger with her for deserting him, in other words to return to the first phase of mourning with all its ambivalence of feeling which at the time of the loss had either been omitted or scamped. The experience of many analysts, well illustrated in a paper by Root (1957), suggests that it is in fact only in this way that such a person can be restored to a life of feeling and attachment.

Strong support for this hypothesis comes from our observations of young children separated from their mothers and unvisited, especially from what we know of the early stages of detachment that follow protest and despair. Once a separated child has entered the phase of detachment he seems no longer preoccupied with his missing mother and instead to have adapted satisfactorily in his new surroundings. When his mother comes to fetch him, so far from greeting her he seems hardly to know her and, so far from clinging to her, remains remote and unresponsive; it is a condition that most mothers find distressing and incomprehensible. Provided the separation has not lasted too long, however, it is reversible, and it is in what happens after reversal that special interest lies.

After a child has been back with his mother a few hours or a few days, the detached behaviour is replaced not only by all the old attachment but by attachment of greatly heightened intensity. From this it is clear that during detachment the ties binding him to his mother have not quietly faded, as is suggested by Anna Freud (1960),* nor has there been a simple forgetting. On the contrary, the data show that during the phase of detachment the responses that bind the child to his mother and lead him to strive to recover her are subject to a defensive process. In some way they are removed from consciousness, but remain latent and ready to become active again, at high intensity, when circumstances change.† This means that in infants and young children the experience of separation habitually initiates defensive processes which lead to yearning for the lost person and reproach for desertion both becoming unconscious. Another way of stating it is that, in early childhood, loss is responded to by processes of mourning that habitually take a course that in adults is deemed pathological.

* In an earlier publication (Burlingham and Freud 1942), however, Anna Freud adopted a viewpoint similar to that taken here.
† The change of circumstance required varies with the stage to which detachment has progressed. When the child is still in the early phases, renewed attachment usually follows reunion with his mother: when he is in an advanced stage analytic treatment is likely to be required.

The question that now arises is whether the defensive processes that are so striking following loss in childhood are different in kind from what is seen in healthy mourning or whether they occur in healthy mourning also but with some difference of form or timing. Evidence suggests that they do occur (Bowlby 1961b), but that in the healthy process their onset is delayed. As a result the urges to recover the lost person and to reproach him or her have time enough for expression so that, through repeated failure, they are gradually relinquished or, in terms of learning theory, extinguished. What appears to happen in childhood (and in the pathological mourning of later years), on the other hand, is that the development of defensive processes is accelerated. As a result, the urges to recover and to reproach the lost person have no chance to be extinguished and instead persist, with consequences that are serious.

Let us return briefly to apply these ideas to Helene Deutsch's patient. Following his mother's death when he was five, it seems, both longing and anger had disappeared from his conscious self. The fantasy of the visit from the dog shows, however, that they persisted none the less at an unconscious level. This and evidence from other cases suggests that, although immobilized, both his love and his anger had remained directed towards the recovery of his dead mother. Thus, locked in the service of a hopeless cause, they had been lost to the developing personality. With loss of mother had gone loss also of his feeling life.

Two common technical terms are in use to denote the processes at work: fixation and repression. Unconsciously the child remains fixated on his lost mother: his urges to recover and to reproach her, and the ambivalent emotions connected with them, have undergone repression.

Another defensive process, closely related to and alternative to repression, can also occur following loss. This is 'splitting of the ego' (Freud 1938). In such cases one part of the personality, secret but conscious, denies that the person is really lost and maintains, instead, either that there is still communication with him or her or that he or she will soon be recovered; whilst simultaneously another part of the personality shares with friends and relatives the knowledge that the person is irretrievably lost. Incompatible though they be, the two parts may coexist over many years. As in the case of repression, ego-splits lead also to psychiatric illness.

Why in some cases the part still yearning to recover the lost person should be conscious and in others it should be unconscious is not clear. Neither are the conditions which lead some bereaved children to develop satisfactorily whilst others do not.[6] This is a problem being studied by Hilgard (Hilgard, Newman, and Fisk 1960). What seems certain, however, is that the precipitate onset of the defensive processes, repression or splitting, with the resulting fixation, is initiated much more readily in childhood than in more mature years. In this fact lies a main explanation, I suggest, of why and how it is that experiences of loss in early childhood lead to faulty personality development and proneness to psychiatric illness.

The hypothesis I am advancing, therefore, is that in the young child the experience of separation from the mother-figure is especially apt to evoke psychological processes of a kind that are as crucial for psychopathology as are inflammation and its resulting scar tissue to physiopathology. This does not mean that a crippling of personality is the inevitable result; but it does mean that, as in the case, say, of rheumatic fever, scar tissue is all too often formed which in later life leads to more or less severe dysfunction. The processes in question, it seems, are pathological variants of those that characterize healthy mourning.

Although this is a theoretical position that is closely akin to many others already in the field, it appears none the less to be different to them. Its strength lies in relating the pathological responses with which we are confronted in older patients to responses to loss that are actually to be observed in early childhood, thereby providing a more solid link between psychiatric conditions of later life and childhood experience. Let us turn now to compare this formulation with some of its predecessors.

TWO TRADITIONS IN PSYCHOANALYTIC THEORIZING

During this century a number of psychoanalysts and psychiatrists have sought to relate together psychiatric illness, loss of a loved person, pathological mourning, and childhood experience. Almost all have taken as their starting-point the sick patient.

It is more than sixty years since Freud first adumbrated the idea that both hysteria and melancholia are manifestations of pathological mourning following more or less recent bereavement (Freud 1954), and more than forty since in *Mourning and Melancholia* he advanced the hypothesis in a systematic way (Freud 1917). Since then there have been a host of other studies all of which in different ways support it.[7] Clinical experience and a reading of the evidence leaves little doubt of the truth of the main proposition – that much psychiatric illness is an expression of pathological mourning – or that such illness includes many cases of anxiety state, depressive illness, and hysteria, and also more than one kind of character disorder. Plainly there has been discovered here a large and important field: for it to be explored fully much further work is required.

Controversy begins when we come to consider why some individuals and not others respond to loss in these pathological ways: and it is amongst hypotheses that seek to account for the origin of such differential responsiveness that the one I am advancing belongs.

An hypothesis that has influenced all later workers with a psychological orientation was outlined by Abraham (1924). As a result of analysing several melancholic patients, he came to the conclusion that 'in the last resort melancholic depression is derived from disagreeable experiences in the childhood of the patient'. He therefore postulated that, during their childhood, melancholics have suffered from what he termed a 'primal parathymia'. In these passages, however, Abraham never used the words grief and mourning; nor is it clear that he recognized that for the young child the experience of losing mother (or of losing her love) is in very truth a bereavement.

Since then, a number of other psychoanalysts in trying to trace the childhood roots of depressive illness and of personalities prone to develop it have drawn attention to unhappy experiences in the early years of their patients' lives. Except in the tradition of theorizing initiated by Melanie Klein, however, few have conceptualized the experiences in terms of bereavement and pathological mourning. Nevertheless, when we come to study the experiences to which they refer, it seems evident that this is the frame of reference that best fits them. I will give as examples three patients described in the literature.

In 1936 Gerö reported two patients suffering from depression. One of them, he concluded, had been 'starved of love' as a child; the other had been sent to a residential nursery and had only returned home when he was three. Each showed intense ambivalence towards any person that was loved, a condition that Gerö believed, could be traced to the early experience. In the second case, he speaks of both a fixation on the mother and an inability to forgive her for the separation. Edith Jacobson in her extensive writing on the psychopathology of depression draws regularly on a female patient, Peggy, whose analysis she describes in two papers (1943, 1946). On referral, Peggy, aged twenty-four, was in a state of severe depression with suicidal impulses and depersonalization; these symptoms had been precipitated by a loss, actually the loss of her lover. The childhood experience on which Edith Jacobson places major emphasis occurred when Peggy was three and a half years old. At this time her mother went to hospital to have a new baby, whilst she and her father stayed with the maternal grandmother. Quarrels developed and father departed. 'The child was left alone, disappointed by her father and eagerly awaiting her mother's return. However, when the mother did return it was with the baby.' Peggy recalled feeling at this time 'This was not my mother, it was a different person' (a feeling that we know is not uncommon in young children who have been separated from their mothers for a few weeks). It was soon after this, Edith Jacobson believed, that 'the little girl broke down in her first deep depression'.

Now it may be questioned both whether the happenings in these patients' early childhoods were accurately recalled and also whether the analysis were right in attributing to them so much significance for their patients' emotional development. But, if we accept as I am inclined to do both the validity of the events and their significance,* I believe the concept of pathological mourning to be the one best fitted to describe both how the patient responded at the time and also to relate the event of childhood to the psychiatric illness of adult life. Neither author utilizes this concept, however. Instead both use concepts such as 'disappointment' and 'disillusionment' which appear to have a different significance.

Several other analysts, whilst in greater or less degree alive to the pathogenic role of such events in childhood, also do not identify the child's response to loss with mourning. One is Fairbairn (1952). A second is Stengel who, in his studies of compulsive wandering (1939, 1941, 1943), draws special attention to the urge to recover the lost object. A third is myself in my earlier work (Bowlby 1944, 1951). Others are Anna Freud (1960) and Rene Spitz (1946), both of whom, by disputing the

---

* In the case of Peggy there is reason to believe that the separation at three and a half was only the culmination in a series of disturbances in her relation to her mother, who is described as a dominating woman who disciplined the child severely.

notion that infants and young children mourn, have ruled out as a possibility the hypothesis that neurotic and psychotic character developments are sometimes the result of mourning in childhood having taken a pathological course.

A main reason why a child's response to loss is so often not identified with mourning appears to be a tradition that confines the concept 'mourning' to processes that have a healthy outcome. Although this usage, like any other, is legitimate, it has one grave disadvantage: logically it becomes impossible to discuss, as such, any variants of mourning that may seem pathological.

The difficulties to which this usage gives rise are illustrated in Helene Deutsch's paper 'Absence of Grief' (1937), from which the case has already been quoted. In her discussion there is firm recognition both of the central place of childhood loss in the production of symptoms and character deviations and also of a defence mechanism which, following loss, may lead to an absence of affect. Nevertheless, although she relates this mechanism to mourning, it is represented more as an alternative to than as a pathological variant of mourning. Whilst at first sight this distinction may appear one merely of terminology, it is of more significance. For to regard the defensive process following childhood loss as an alternative to mourning is to miss both that defensive processes of similar kinds but of lesser degree and later onset enter also into healthy mourning, and also that what is pathological is not so much the defensive processes themselves as their intensity and the prematurity of their onset.

Similarly, although Freud was on the one hand deeply interested in the pathogenic role of mourning and on the other, especially in his later years, was also aware of the pathogenic role of childhood loss, he seems none the less never to have put his finger on childhood mourning and its disposition to take a pathological course as concepts which link these two sets of ideas together. This is well illustrated in his discussion of the splitting of the ego in the defensive process, to which he was giving special attention at the end of his life (1938).

In one of his papers on the subject (1927), Freud describes two patients in whom an ego-split had followed loss of father. 'In the analysis of two young men,' he writes, 'I learnt that each of them – one in his second and the other in his tenth year – had refused to acknowledge the death of his father . . . and yet neither of them had developed a psychosis. A very important piece of reality had thus been denied by the ego . . .' But, he continues, 'it was only one current of their mental processes that had not acknowledged the father's death; there was another that was fully aware of the fact; the one which was consistent with reality [namely that the father was dead] stood alongside the one which accorded with a wish' [that the father should still be living] (1927). In this and related papers, however, Freud does not relate his discovery of such splits in the ego to the pathology of mourning in general nor to childhood mourning in particular. He did recognize them, nevertheless, as the not uncommon sequelae of bereavements sustained in early life. 'I suspect', he remarks when discussing his findings, 'that similar occurrences are by no means rare in childhood.' Recent statistical studies, we find, show that his suspicion was well founded.

Thus a reading of the literature shows that, despite attributing much pathogenic significance to loss of a parent and to loss of love, in the main tradition of psychoanalytic theorizing the origin of pathological mourning and of the consequent psychiatric illness in the adult is not connected with the disposition for processes of mourning to take a pathological course when they occur following a loss in infancy and early childhood.

I believe it to have been a major contribution of Melanie Klein (1935, 1940), to have made this connection. Infants and young children mourn and go through phases of depression, she maintains, and their modes of responding at such times are determinants of the way that in later life they will respond to further loss. Certain methods of defence, she believes, are to be understood as 'directed against the "pining" for the lost object'. In these respects my approach is similar to her's. Differences arise, however, over the particular events that are thought to be of importance, the age at which they are thought to occur, and the nature and origin of anxiety and aggression.

The losses that Melanie Klein has suggested are pathogenic all belong to the first year of life and are mostly connected with feeding and weaning. Aggression is regarded as an expression of the death instinct, and anxiety the result of its projection. I find none of this convincing. In the first place the evidence she advances regarding the overwhelming importance of the first year and of weaning is, on scrutiny, far from impressive (Bowlby 1960b). In the second, her hypotheses regarding aggression and anxiety are not easy to fit into a framework of biological theory (Bowlby 1960a). It is, I believe, because so many find the elaborations with which Melanie Klein has surrounded the hypothesis regarding the role of childhood mourning implausible that the hypothesis itself remains neglected. This is a pity.

My position therefore is that, although I do not regard the details of Melanie Klein's theory of the depressive position as a satisfactory way of accounting for why individuals develop in such diverse ways that some respond to later loss with healthy mourning whilst others do so with one or another form of pathological mourning, I none the less hold her theory to contain the seeds of a very productive way of ordering the data. The alternative elaborations which I believe the evidence favours are that the most significant object that can be lost is not the breast but the mother herself (and sometimes the father), that the vulnerable period is not confined to the first year but extends over a number of years of childhood (as Freud (1938) himself held), and that loss of a parent gives rise not only to primary separation anxiety and grief but to processes of mourning in which aggression, the function of which is to achieve reunion, plays a major part. Whilst sticking closely to the data, this formulation has the additional merit of fitting readily into biological theory.

Substantial though the differences are between Melanie Klein's standpoint and mine, the area of agreement is also substantial. Both hold as a main hypothesis that processes of mourning occurring in these early years are more apt than when they occur later in life to take a pathological course and so to leave the individual thenceforward more prone than others to respond to further loss in a similar way. The version of this theory that I am now advancing appears to be consistent with much of the clinical material published in the literature and already referred to. This includes Freud's cases of splits in the ego, Stengel's cases of compulsive wandering, the depressive patients described by Abraham, Gerö, and Edith Jacobson, and the patients with character defects described by Helene Deutsch, Melanie Klein, Fairbairn and myself. It is also consistent with the numerous studies that have appeared in the past two decades that show that the incidence of childhood loss in the lives of patients suffering from psychiatric illness and character defect is significantly higher than it is for the general population. [Since statistical data up to 1967 are presented in the next Lecture those in the original version of this one have been omitted. Some of the commentary is retained, however.]

Nevertheless, in considering the relevance of the statistical data to my argument certain doubts are likely to arise. In the first place we must beware of the fallacy *post hoc ergo propter hoc*. In the second, even if we are right in claiming a casual relationship between early loss and subsequent illness, it does not follow that it is always mediated by means of the pathological processes that have been described earlier. There are, indeed, two other sorts of process which almost certainly give rise to pathology in some cases. One is the process of identification with parents, which is an integral part of healthy development but which often leads to difficulties after one of them has died.* The other sort are evoked by the surviving parent, widow or widower, whose attitude towards the child may change and become pathogenic.

There is another difficulty that the hypothesis must meet. Even if it is true that there is an increased incidence of death of parents in the childhood histories of individuals prone later to develop certain types of personality and certain forms of illness, its absolute incidence is nevertheless low. How, it will be asked, are the other cases to be accounted for? There is more than one possible explanation.

In the first place, in order to base my argument on firm evidence, I have deliberately restricted most of the discussion to the incidence of parental *death*. When other causes of parental loss in the early years are included the percentage of cases affected is greatly increased. Furthermore, for many of the cases in which there has been no episode of actual separation in space of child from parent, there is often evidence that there has none the less been separation of another and more or less serious kind. Rejection, loss of love (perhaps on advent of a new baby or on account of mother's depression), alienation from one parent by the other, and similar situations, all have as a common factor loss by the child of a parent to love and to attach himself to. If the concept of loss is extended to cover loss of love these cases no longer constitute exceptions.

It seems unlikely, however, that such an extension would cover all cases falling within the psychiatric syndromes concerned. If this proves to be so some other explanation for those not accounted for by the present hypothesis needs to be sought. Perhaps on closer examination the clinical picture of such cases

---

* Psychiatric disturbance in which identification with a lost parent plays a significant part has for long been a subject of study by analysts. It is particularly clear in anniversary reactions (Hilgard and Newman 1959).

will prove to be different in material degree to those that are accounted for. Alternatively, the clinical conditions may prove to be essentially similar but the pathological processes at work in cases not accounted for to have been initiated by events of a different kind. Until these and other possibilities have been explored problems will remain. Since, however, there is rarely a simple relationship between syndrome, pathological process, and pathogenic experience, the problems are no different to those that occur constantly in other fields of medical research.

CONCLUSION

It is probable that by far the most research in the field of psychiatry today still starts with an end-product, a sick patient, and seeks to unravel the sequence of events, psychological and physiological, that appear to have led to his becoming sick. This results in many suggestive hypotheses but, like any single method of inquiry, has its limitations. One of the hallmarks of an advancing science is exploitation of as many methods as can be devised. When in physiological medicine research was expanded to include the systematic investigation of one or another probable pathogen and its effects, a great harvest of knowledge was garnered. Perhaps the day is not far distant when the same will be possible in psychiatry.

Because of its practical and scientific implications, the study of responses to loss of mother-figure in the early years is of promise. On the practical side there is likelihood of our becoming able to develop measures to prevent at least some forms of mental ill health. On the scientific side there are opportunities that stem from the identification of an event of childhood that is probably pathogenic, can be clearly defined, and the effects of which on the developing personality can be systematically studied by direct observation.

There are, of course, many other events of childhood besides loss that there is good reason to believe also contribute to the development of disturbed personality and psychiatric illness. Examples are the child's being exposed to one or another of the various sorts of parental attitude that have long been the subject of concern and therapeutic endeavour in child psychiatric clinics. For each the research task is, first, to define the event or sequence of events, second, to locate a sample of cases in which it is occurring so that its effects on psychological development may be studied, and, finally, to relate the processes that are found to be set in train by it to processes present in patients with declared illness. The consequences of such an expansion of research are far-reaching.

NOTES

1   In the original version of this lecture I referred to a change in the 'strength' of attachment. To think of attachment as varying according to its strength, however, has proved extremely misleading and has been abandoned by informed workers. Often it is useful to think of attachment as varying along a dimension 'secure-anxious'. See my discussion in the opening paragraphs of Chapter 15 of *Attachment and Loss*, Volume 2.

2   See especially the work reported by Heinicke and Westheimer (1966), some of the findings from which are given in Chapter 4.

3   In the original version of this lecture (and in a few places in the previous two) I followed the psychoanalytic tradition of referring to 'object relations', 'the loved object', and 'the lost object'. Shortly afterwards I abandoned this usage. Not only does it stem from a theoretical paradigm that even in 1961 I no longer favoured, but I regard it as seriously misleading to refer to another person as an object since it implies that the relationship is with something inert instead of with another human being who plays an equal or perhaps a dominant part in determining how the relationship develops. In republishing this lecture, therefore, I have changed the wording and refer throughout to a 'loved person' or 'lost person' instead of to 'loved object' or 'lost object'.

4   It is now clear that mourning processes in children need not take a

course that leads to pathology, though they all too often do. The adjective 'habitually' used in the text here and elsewhere in this lecture is therefore misleading. The conditions influencing outcome are discussed by Furman (1974) and are dealt with in some detail also in Part III of *Attachment and Loss*, Volume 3.

5   Not infrequently the reasons for a child failing to respond with feeling to a parent's death is that he is given little or no information about what has happened and, even if he is informed, is given no opportunity to express his feelings or to ask questions of a sympathetic adult. For references see note 4 above.

6   Much more is now known about the relevant conditions; see notes 4 and 5 above.

7   See especially the books by Parkes (1972) and Glick, Weiss, and Parkes (1974).

4

EFFECTS ON BEHAVIOUR OF DISRUPTION OF AN AFFECTIONAL BOND*

For a number of years the Eugenics Society organized symposia dealing with the interaction of genetic and environmental factors in human development. The fourth symposium, held in London during the autumn of 1967, was concerned with 'Genetic and Environmental Influences on Behaviour'. The paper that follows was a contribution to the symposium, which was published the following year.

Family doctors, priests, and perceptive laymen have long been aware that there are few blows to the human spirit so great as the loss of someone near and dear. Traditional wisdom knows that we can be crushed by grief and die of a broken heart, and also

* Originally published in Thoday, J. M. and Parker, A. S. (eds.) (1968) *Genetic and Environmental Influences on Behaviour*. Edinburgh: Oliver & Boyd. Reprinted by permission of The Eugenics Society.

that a jilted lover is apt to do things that are foolish or dangerous to himself and others. It knows too that neither love nor grief is felt for just *any* other human being, but only for one, or a few, particular and individual human beings. The core of what I term an 'affectional bond' is the attraction that one *individual* has for another *individual*.

Until recent decades, science has had little to say about these matters. Experimental scientists in the physiological or Hullian learning theory traditions of psychology have never shown interest in affectional bonds, and have sometimes talked and acted as though they do not exist. Psychoanalysts, by contrast, have long recognized the immense importance of affectional bonds in the lives and problems of their patients, but they have been slow to develop an adequate scientific framework within which the formation, maintenance, and disruption of such bonds can be understood. The void has been filled by ethologists, starting with Lorenz's classical paper on *The Companion in the Bird's World* (1935), progressing through a multitude of experiments on imprinting (Bateson 1966; Sluckin 1964) to studies of bonding behaviour in non-human primates (Hinde and Spencer-Booth 1967; Sade 1965) and inspiring psychologists to make similar studies of humans (Ainsworth 1967; Schaffer and Emerson 1964).

PREVALENCE OF BONDING

Before discussing the effects of bond disruption a note about bonding and its prevalence is in place. The work referred to shows that, even if not universal in birds and mammals, strong and persistent bonds between individuals are the rule in very many species. The types of bond that are made differ from one species to another, the commonest being those between one or both parents and their offspring and those between adults of opposite sex. In mammals, including the primates, the first and most persistent bond of all is usually that between mother and young, a bond which often persists into adult life. As a result of all this work, it is now possible to view the strong and persistent affectional bonds made by humans from a comparative stand-point.

Affectional bonding is a result of the social behaviour of each individual of a species, differing according to which other individual of his species he is dealing with; which entails of course an ability to recognize individuals. Whilst each member of a bonded pair tends both to remain in proximity to the other and to elicit proximity-keeping behaviour in the other, individuals who are not bonded show no such tendencies; indeed, when two individuals are not bonded, one often strongly resists any approach the other may attempt. Examples are the attitudes of a parent towards the approach of young not its own, and of a male towards the approach of another male.

The essential feature of affectional bonding is that the two partners tend to remain in proximity to one another. Should they for any reason be apart, each will sooner or later seek out the other and so renew proximity. Any attempt by a third party to separate a bonded pair is strenuously resisted: not infrequently the stronger of the partners attacks the intruder whilst the weaker flees, or perhaps clings to the stronger partner. Obvious examples are situations in which an intruder is attempting to remove young from a mother, e.g., calf from cow, or to detach the female from a bonded heterosexual pair, e.g., goose from gander.

A little paradoxically, behaviour of an aggressive sort plays a key role in maintaining affectional bonds. It takes two distinct forms: first, attacks on and frightening away of intruders and, second, the punishment of an errant partner, be it wife, husband, or child. There is evidence that much aggressive behaviour of a puzzling and pathological kind originates in one or other of these ways (Bowlby 1963).

Affectional bonds and subjective states of strong emotion tend to go together, as every novelist and playwright knows. Thus, many of the most intense of all human emotions arise during the formation, the maintenance, the disruption, and the renewal of affectional bonds – which, for that reason, are sometimes called emotional bonds. In terms of subjective experience, the formation of a bond is described as falling in love, maintaining a bond as loving someone, and losing a partner as grieving over someone. Similarly, threat of loss arouses anxiety and actual loss causes sorrow; whilst both situations are likely to arouse anger. Finally, the unchallenged maintenance of a bond is experienced as a source of security, and the renewal of a bond as a source of joy. Thus, anyone concerned with the psychology and psycho-pathology of emotion, whether in animals or man, is soon confronted by problems of affectional bonding: what causes bonds to develop and what they are there for, and especially the conditions that affect the form their development takes.

In so far as psychologists and psychoanalysts have attempted to account for the existence of affectional bonds, the motives of food and sex have almost always been invoked. Thus in attempting to explain why a child becomes attached to his mother, both learning theorists (Dollard and Miller 1950; Sears, Maccoby, and Levin 1957) and psychoanalysts (Freud 1938) have independently assumed that it is because mother *feeds* child. In attempting to understand why adults become attached to one another, sex has commonly been seen as the obvious and sufficient explanation. Yet, once the evidence is scrutinized, these explanations are found wanting. There is now abundant evidence that, not only in birds but in mammals also, young become attached to mother-objects despite not being fed from that source (Harlow and Harlow 1965; Cairns 1966) and that by no means all affectional bonding between adults is accompanied by sexual relations; whereas, conversely, sexual relations often occur independently of any persisting affectional bonds.

What is now known of the ontogeny of affectional bonds suggests that they develop because the young creature is born with a strong bias to approach certain classes of stimuli, notably the familiar, and to avoid other classes, notably the strange. As regards function, observation of animals in the wild strongly suggests that the biological function of much, if not all, bonding is protection from predators – a function fully as important for the survival of a population as nutrition or reproduction, but one which has habitually been overlooked by workers confined in laboratories and concerned only with man living in economically developed societies.

Whether these hypotheses are supported by further work or not, an individual's capacity to make affectional bonds of a type appropriate to each phase of his species' life cycle and to his or her own sex is plainly a capacity as typical of individuals of mammalian species as are their capacities, for example, to see, to hear, to eat, and to digest. And in all likelihood a capacity for bonding has as high a survival value to a species as has any of these other long-studied capacities. It is proving productive to view many of the psychoneurotic and personality disturbances of humans as being a reflection of a disturbed capacity for making affectional bonds, due either to faulty development during childhood or to subsequent derangement.

DISRUPTED BONDS AND PSYCHIATRIC ILLNESS

Those who suffer from psychiatric disturbances, whether psychoneurotic, sociopathic, or psychotic, always show impairment of the capacity for affectional bonding, an impairment that is often both severe and long lasting. Although in some cases this impairment is clearly secondary to other changes, in many it is probably primary and derives from faulty development having occurred during a childhood spent in an atypical family environment. Whilst disruption of the bonds that tie a child to his parents is not the only form, adverse in this respect, that the environment can take, it is the form most reliably recorded and the effects of which we know most about.*

In considering the possible causes of psychiatric disturbance in childhood, child psychiatrists were early aware that antecedent conditions of significantly high incidence are either an absence of opportunity to make affectional bonds or else long and perhaps repeated disruptions of bonds once made (Bowlby 1951; Ainsworth 1962). Though the view that such conditions are not only associated with subsequent disturbance but are causal of it is widely held, that conclusion nevertheless remains debatable.

Studies of the incidence of childhood loss in different samples of psychiatric populations have multiplied in recent years. Due to the samples and the comparison groups being so differently constituted, to criteria of loss being differently defined, and to a host of demographical and statistical hazards, their interpretation is not easy. Certain findings, however, have been so consistently reported by independent workers, including reports of a number of recent and well-controlled studies, that we can be reasonably confident of them. Two psychiatric syndromes and two sorts of associated symptom are consistently found to be preceded by a high incidence of disrupted affectional bonds during childhood. The syndromes are psychopathic (or sociopathic) personality and depression; the symptoms persistent delinquency and suicide.

The *psychopath* (or *sociopath*) is a person who, whilst not being psychotic or mentally subnormal, persistently engages in: (i) acts against society, e.g., crime; (ii) acts against the family, e.g., neglect, cruelty, sexual promiscuity, or perversion; (iii) acts

---

* There are also valuable studies of the reaction of adults to bereavement and of the relationship of bereavement reactions to mental illness (Parkes 1965). In a short paper it has not been possible to include discussion of these findings.

against himself, e.g., addiction, suicide, or attempted suicide, repeatedly abandoning his job.

In such people the capacity to make and maintain affectional bonds is always disordered and not infrequently conspicuous by its absence.

More often than not the childhoods of such individuals are found to have been grossly disturbed by the death, divorce, or separation of the parents, or by other events resulting in disruption of bonds, with an incidence of such disturbance far higher than is met with in any other comparable group, whether drawn from the general population or from psychiatric casualties of other sorts. For example, in a study of well over a thousand consecutive psychiatric out-patients under the age of sixty, Earle and Earle (1961) diagnosed sixty-six as sociopaths and 1357 as suffering from some other disorder. Taking as their criterion an absence of mother for six months or more before the sixth birthday, Earle and Earle found an incidence of 41 per cent for the sociopaths and 5 per cent for the remainder.

When the criterion is made broader the incidence rises. Thus Craft, Stephenson, and Granger (1964) took as their criterion an absence of either mother or father (or both) before the child's tenth birthday. Of seventy-six male inmates of the special hospitals for aggressive psychopaths, no less than 65 per cent had had such an experience. In a study of several comparison groups Craft shows how the incidence of this type of childhood experience rises with the degree of antisocial behaviour shown by a group's members.

Others who have reported similar sorts of statistically significant findings for groups of psychopaths and persistent delinquents are Naess (1962), Greer (1964a), and Brown and Epps (1966); and for alcoholics and addicts, Dennehy (1966).

In psychopaths the incidence of illegitimacy and a shunting of the child from one 'home' to another is high. It is no accident that Brady of the 'Moors' murders was such a one.

Another psychiatric group which shows a much increased incidence of childhood loss is that of *suicidal patients*, both those who attempt suicide and those who succeed.* The losses are especially likely to have occurred during the first five years of life and to have been caused not only by the death of a parent, but also by other long-lasting causes, notably illegitimacy and divorce. In these respects suicidal patients tend to resemble sociopaths and, as will be seen later, to differ from depressives.

Of the many studies reporting a very high incidence of childhood loss among attempted suicides, e.g., Bruhn (1962), Greer (1964b), and Kessel (1965), a recent study by Greer, Gunn, and Koller (1966) is amongst the best-controlled. A series of 156 attempted suicides were compared with similar-sized samples of non-suicidal psychiatric patients and of surgical and obstetric patients without a psychiatric history; both comparison groups were matched with the attempted suicides in respect of age, sex, class, and other relevant variables. Taking as his criterion of loss the continuous absence of one or both parents for at least twelve months, Greer finds that such events have occurred before the fifth birthday three times as often in the group of attempted suicides as in either of the comparison groups – an incidence of 26 per cent against 9 per cent for each of the others (*Table 1*).

Furthermore, the losses in the attempted suicide group tended more often to have been of both parents and to have been permanent, whereas in the other groups they more often concerned only one parent and were temporary, having been due to such exigencies as illness or work.[1]

---

* Although any group of suicides and attempted suicides will contain some sociopaths and some depressives, a majority are likely to be diagnosed as suffering from neurosis or personality disorder (Greer, Gunn, and Koller 1966) and so constitute a fairly distinct psychiatric group.

Table 1 Incidence of loss or continuous absence of one or both natural parents for at least 12 months before the 15th birthday

	Non-psychiatric patients %	Non-suicidal psychiatric patients %	Attempted suicide %
age at loss			
0–4 years	9	9	26
5–9 years	12	10	11
10–14 years	7	7	11
doubtful	0	2	1
0–14	28	28	49
N	156	156	156

In a further study of the same group of attempted suicides (Greer and Gunn 1966) it was found that those who had suffered parental loss before their fifteenth birthday differed significantly in certain respects from those who had not. One such difference, in keeping with other findings, is that those who had suffered childhood loss were more likely to be diagnosed as sociopaths than were those who had not suffered a childhood loss (18 per cent against 4 per cent).

Another condition which is associated with a significantly increased incidence of childhood loss is depression. The type of loss experienced, however, tends to be of a kind different to the overall family disruption typical of the childhoods of psychopaths and attempted suicides. First, in the childhoods of depressives loss is more often due to the death of a parent than to illegitimacy, divorce, or separation. Second, in depressives the incidence of bereavement tends to be increased during the second quinquennium of childhood, and in some studies also the third. Findings of this sort have been reported by F. Brown (1961), Munro (1966), Dennehy (1966), and Hill and Price

(1967). Indications are that loss of a parent by death occurs about twice as frequently in a group of depressives as it does in the population as a whole.[2]

Thus, it now seems reasonably certain that in several groups of psychiatric patients the incidence of disruption of affectional bonds during childhood is significantly raised. Whilst these later studies confirm the earlier findings regarding the increased incidence of loss of mother during early childhood, they also extend them. For several sorts of condition increased incidences of disrupted bonds are now seen to include bonds to fathers as well as to mothers, and to be found during the years from five to fourteen as well as during the first five. Furthermore, in the more extreme conditions, sociopathy and suicidal tendencies, not only is an initial loss likely to have occurred early in life but it is likely also to have been both a permanent loss and to have been followed by the child experiencing repeated shifts of parent figures.

Nevertheless, to demonstrate an increased incidence of some factor is only one thing: to demonstrate that it plays a causal role is quite another. Whilst most of those reporting the findings referred to believe that the increased incidence of childhood loss bears a causal relation to the subsequent psychiatric disturbance, and there is a wealth of clinical records pointing in that direction (for references see Bowlby 1963), alternative explanations still remain possible. As an example, the increased incidence of maternal and paternal death in psychiatric patients might be a result of the parents of patients being older than average at the time of the patient's birth. Were this so, not only would early death of a parent be more likely but there might also be greater liability for the offspring to be born with an adverse genetic loading. Thus, what appears to be an environmental determinant might turn out to be a genetic one after all.

To test that possibility is not easy. For it to be supported requires: first, that the mean ages of the mothers and/or fathers of psychiatric patients be found in fact to be higher than the means for the population as a whole; and, second, that any increased parental age that may be found be shown to have an adverse effect on the genetic endowment of the offspring such that the likelihood of psychiatric disability is increased. The first requirement may well be met: recent evidence (Dennehy 1966) suggests that mean ages of the parents of psychiatric patients may be above those of the population from which they come. The second requirement, however, is more difficult to get evidence about. Plainly it may be some time before the issue is settled.

Meanwhile, those who believe that the relationship between disruption of affectional bonds during childhood and disturbance of the capacity to maintain affectional bonds typical of personality disorders of later life is a causal one point to other evidence in support of their hypothesis. It concerns the way young humans and sub-human primates behave when an affectional bond is broken by separation or death.

SHORT-TERM EFFECTS OF DISRUPTED BONDS

When a young child finds himself with strangers and without his familiar parent figures, not only is he intensely distressed at the time but his subsequent relationship with his parents is impaired, at least temporarily. The behaviour seen in two-year-olds during and after a short stay in a residential nursery is the subject of a systematic descriptive and statistical study undertaken at the Tavistock by Heinicke and Westheimer (1966). The particular part of their report to which I draw attention is that in which they compare the behaviour towards mother of ten children who had been away in the nursery and are now returned home, with that of a comparison group of ten young children who had remained at home throughout.

In the separated children two forms of disturbance of affectional behaviour were seen, neither of which was observed in the comparison group of non-separated children. One form is that of emotional detachment; the other its apparent opposite, namely an unrelenting demand to be close to mother.

(1) On first meeting his mother after he has been away from home with strangers for two or three weeks a two-year-old child typically remains distant and detached. Whereas during his early days away a child commonly cries pathetically for his mother, when at last she returns he seems not to recognize her or avoids her. Instead of rushing to her and clinging as he probably would if he had been lost in a shop for half an hour, he often looks right through her and refuses her hand. All the proximity-seeking behaviour typical of an affectional bond is missing, usually to the mother's intense distress; and it remains missing – sometimes only for minutes or hours but sometimes for days. Resumption of attachment may be sudden, but is often slow and piecemeal. The length of time detachment persists is positively correlated with the length of the separation (Table 2).

(2) When – as is usual – attachment behaviour is resumed, a child is commonly much more clinging than he was before the separation. He dislikes his mother leaving him and tends either

Table 2 Number of separated and non-separated children who showed detachment during first 3 days after reunion (or during equivalent period)

	Separated	Non-separated
no detachment	–	10
detachment for one day only	1	–
detachment alternating with clinging	4	–
detachment persistent for 3 days	5	–
	10	10

Degree of detachment correlated with length of separation: r = 0.82; P = 0.01.

to cry or to follow her round the house. How this phase evolves turns largely on how his mother responds. Not infrequently conflict ensues, a child demanding his mother's constant company and she refusing it. Such refusal readily evokes hostile and negative behaviour from the child, which is apt to try his mother's patience still further. Of the ten separated children observed by Heinicke and Westheimer six showed strong and persistent hostile behaviour to mother and negativism after their return home: no such behaviour was seen in the non-separated children (Table 3).

Clearly it is still a far cry between showing that a child's bonds to his mother, and often to his father also, are thrown into disequilibrium by a brief separation, and demonstrating unequivocally that long or repeated separations are causally related to subsequent personality disorders. Yet the detached behaviour so typical of young children after a separation bears more than a passing resemblance to the detached behaviour of some psychopaths, whilst it would be difficult to distinguish the aggressively demanding behaviour of many a young child recently reunited with his mother from the aggressively demanding behaviour of

Table 3 Number of separated and non-separated children who showed strong and persistent hostility to mother after reunion (or during equivalent period)

	Separated	Non-separated
little or no hostile behaviour or negativism to mother	4	10
strong and persistent hostile behaviour and negativism to mother	6	0
	10 P = 0.01	10

many hysterical personalities. To postulate that in each type of case the disturbed behaviour of the adult represents a persistence over the years of deviant patterns of bonding behaviour that have become established as a result of bond disruptions occurring during childhood proves useful. On the one hand it helps to organize data and to orient further research; on the other it provides guidelines for the day-to-day management of these kinds of people.

To advance our knowledge in this field it would obviously be invaluable to conduct a long series of experiments to investigate the short- and long-term effects on behaviour of disrupting an affectional bond, taking into account the subject's age, the nature of the bond, the length and frequency of disruptions, and many other variables besides. Equally obvious, however, is that any such experiments on human subjects are ruled out on ethical grounds. For these reasons it is much to be welcomed that comparable experiments using non-human primates are now being undertaken. Preliminary findings suggest that the effects on six-month-old rhesus infants of a temporary loss of mother (six days) are, both during and after the separation, not unlike those on two-year-old human children (Spencer-Booth and Hinde 1966), e.g., distress and a lowered level of activity during the separation, and an exceptionally strong tendency to cling to mother after it is over. The monkey-mother's reactions to this, moreover, are not unlike the human mother's. To date, however, there is no record of a monkey baby showing detachment, and this may represent a species difference.

Both in human and in monkey children there are very wide individual variations in the reaction to disruption of a bond. Some of this variation is probably due to the effects on an infant of events occuring during pregnancy and birth. Thus Ucko (1965) found that boys who at birth had been recorded as having been in an asphyxiated state are very much more sensitive to environmental change, including separation from mother, than

Table 4 Distress at temporary separation from mother, father, or sibling in young boys anoxic at birth and non-anoxic at birth

	2nd year		3rd year	
	Distressed	Not	Distressed	Not
anoxic	8	2	9	2
non-anoxic	2	12	4	7
significance	$P = 0.01$		$P = 0.1$	

Total samples comprise 29 pairs of boys matched for class, birth order, and maternal age.

boys who at birth had not been asphyxiated (*Table* 4). Some other part of this variance, on the other hand, may well be genetically determined. Indeed, it is a reasonable hypothesis that a principal way in which genetic factors act to influence the development of mental health and ill-health is by their effect on bonding behaviour: in what degree and form, and in what circumstances, can an individual make and maintain affectional bonds, and how does he respond to disruption of bonds. By undertaking studies of this sort it may in future be possible to bring together environmental and genetic studies of behavioural disorder.

NOTES

1   See also a further study of the relationship between childhood bereavement and ideas of suicide by Adam (1973).

2   Statistical findings in regard to the incidence of parent loss during the childhoods of depressed adults have often been contradictory and I have simplified the original version of this paragraph to bring it into line with current thinking.

     The most recent and comprehensive study of the problem (though confined to women) is that of George Brown and Tirril Harris (1978). They conclude that childhood loss contributes to clinical depression in three distinct ways. First, women who have lost mother by death or separation before the age of eleven are more likely to respond to loss, threatened loss, and other troubles and crises in adult life by developing a depressive disorder than are women without such loss. Second, if a woman has suffered one or more losses of family members by death or separation before the age of seventeen, any depression subsequently developing is likely to be more severe than it would be in a woman without such loss. Third, the form taken by the childhood loss affects the form of any depressive illness that may later develop. When the childhood loss has been due to separation, any illness subsequently developing is likely to show features of neurotic depression, with symptoms of anxiety. When the loss has been due to death, any illness subsequently developing is likely to show features of a psychotic depression, with much retardation.

Brown and Harris also call attention to some of the hitherto unrecognized problems of obtaining valid figures when making comparisons between a group of psychiatrically ill patients and a control group.

5

SEPARATION AND LOSS
WITHIN THE FAMILY*

In the spring of 1968, when I happened to be in California, the San Francisco Psychoanalytic Society organized a conference for mental health workers of all professions on 'Separation and Loss'. I was invited to contribute and presented a version of this paper. It was subsequently amplified with the assistance of my colleague, Colin Murray Parkes, and the result published in 1970 under our joint authorship. It is republished here with his permission.

Probably all of us today are keenly aware of the anxiety and distress that can be caused by separations from loved figures, of the deep and prolonged grief that can follow bereavement, and of the hazards to mental health that these events can constitute. Once eyes are opened, it is seen that many of the troubles we are

* Originally published in Anthony, E. J. and Koupernik, C. (eds.) (1970) The Child in His Family Volume 1. New York: John Wiley. Copyright © 1970 John Wiley & Sons Inc. Reprinted by permission.

called upon to treat in our patients are to be traced, at least in part, to a separation or a loss that occurred either recently or at some earlier period in life. Chronic anxiety, intermittent depression, attempted or successful suicide are some of the more common sorts of troubles that we now know are traceable to such experiences. Furthermore, prolonged or repeated disruptions of the mother-child bond during the first five years of life are known to be especially frequent in patients later diagnosed as psychopathic or sociopathic personalities.

Evidence for these statements, especially that relating to the much increased incidence of loss of a parent during childhood in samples of patients with these troubles when compared to control samples is reviewed elsewhere.* A point we particularly want to emphasize is that, although losses occurring during the first five years are probably especially dangerous for future personality development, losses that occur later in life are potentially pathogenic also.

Although today a causal linkage between psychological disturbance and a separation or loss that occurred at some time during childhood or adolescence, or later, is well attested, both statistically and clinically, there remain very many problems in understanding both the processes at work and also the exact conditions that determine whether outcome is good or bad. Yet, we are not wholly ignorant. Our plan in this paper is to give special attention to the ways in which we may be able to help our patients. Whether they are young or old, and whether the loss is recent or long passed, we believe we can now discern certain principles on which to base our therapy.

We shall start by describing grief and mourning as they occur in adults and work thence to childhood.

* [Namely Chapters 3 and 4 in this volume.]

GRIEF AND MOURNING IN ADULT LIFE

There is now a good deal of reliable information about the way in which adults respond to a major bereavement. It stems from a number of sources, notably the records of Lindemann (1944) and Marris (1958), amplified by a recent and still largely unpublished study (Parkes 1969, 1971b).* Though the intensity of grief varies considerably from individual to individual and the length of each phase also varies, there is none the less a basic overall pattern.

In an earlier paper (Bowlby 1961b), it was suggested that the course of mourning could be divided into three main phases, but we realize now that this numbering omitted an important first phase, which is usually fairly brief. What were formerly numbered phases 1, 2, and 3 have therefore been renumbered phases 2, 3, and 4. The four phases now recognized are:

1. Phase of numbness that usually lasts from a few hours to a week and may be interrupted by outbursts of extremely intense distress and/or anger.
2. Phase of yearning and searching for the lost figure, lasting some months and often for years.
3. Phase of disorganization and despair.
4. Phase of greater or less degree of reorganization.

* Information was obtained from a fairly representative sample of twenty-two widows between the ages of twenty-six and sixty-five during the year following loss of a husband. Each widow was given not less than five long clinical interviews at 1, 3, 6, 9, and 12½ months after bereavement. Good rapport was obtained, and much gratitude was expressed for the understanding given. In ten cases the husband's death had been sudden; in three it was rapid; and in nine it had been foreseen by at least a week.

Phase of numbing

The immediate reaction to news of a husband's death in our study varied very greatly among the widows and also from time to time in any widow. Most felt stunned and in varying degrees quite unable to accept the news. A case in which the phase lasted rather longer than usual was that of a widow who reported that, when told of her husband's death, she had remained calm and 'felt nothing at all' – and was therefore surprised to find herself crying. She consciously avoided her feelings, she said, because she feared she would be overcome or go insane. For three weeks she continued controlled and relatively composed, until finally she broke down in the street and wept. Reflecting on those three weeks, she later described them as having been like 'walking on the edge of a black pit'.

Many other widows reported how the news had altogether failed to register with them at first. Nevertheless, this calm before the storm was sometimes broken by an outburst of extreme emotion, usually of fearfulness, but often of anger, and in one or two cases of elation.

Phase of yearning and searching for the lost figure

Within days or a week or two of the loss a change occurs and the bereaved begins, though only episodically, to register the reality of the loss: this leads to spasms of intense distress and tearfulness. Yet, almost at the same time, there is great restlessness, preoccupation with thoughts of the lost person combined often with a sense of his actual presence, and a marked tendency to interpret signals or sounds as indicating that the lost person is now returned. For example, hearing a door latch lifted at 5 p.m. is interpreted as husband returning from work, or a man in the street is misperceived as the missing husband.

Some or all of these features were found to occur in the great majority of the widows interviewed. Since the same features are also reported by several other investigators, there can be no doubt that they are a regular feature of grief and in no sense abnormal.

When evidence of this sort was reviewed some years ago (Bowlby 1961b), the view was advanced that during this phase of mourning the bereaved is seized by an urge to search for and to recover the lost figure. Sometimes the person is conscious of this urge, though often he is not: sometimes a person willingly falls in with it, as when he visits the grave or visits other places closely linked with the lost figure, but sometimes he seeks to stifle it as irrational and absurd. Whatever the attitude a person may take towards this urge, however, he none the less finds himself impelled to search and, if possible, to recover.

This view was advanced in 1961. So far as we know, it has not been called in question, though we doubt whether it is yet widely accepted. However that may be, the further evidence now available shows it to be well supported.

The following is taken from a recent paper in which evidence for the search hypothesis is set out:

> Although we tend to think of searching in terms of the motor act of restless movement toward possible locations of the lost object, [searching] also has perceptual and ideational components . . . Signs of the object can be identified only by reference to memories of the object as it was. Searching the external world for signs of the object therefore includes the establishment of an internal perceptual 'set' derived from previous experience of the object.
>
> (Parkes 1969)

An example is given of a woman searching for her small son who is missing: she moves restlessly about the likely parts of the house scanning with her eyes and thinking of the boy; she hears a creak and immediately identifies it as the sound of her son's footfall on the stair; she calls out, 'John is that you?' The components of this sequence are:

(a) restless moving about and scanning the environment;
(b) thinking intensely about the lost person;
(c) developing a perceptual 'set' for the person, namely a disposition to perceive and to pay attention to any stimuli that suggest the presence of the person and to ignore all those that are not relevant to this aim;
(d) directing attention towards those parts of the environment in which the person is likely to be;
(e) calling for the lost person.

It is emphasized that each of these components is to be found in bereaved men and women; in addition some grievers are consciously aware of an urge to search.

Two very usual features of mourning which were interpreted in our earlier papers as being a part of this urge to search are weeping and anger.

The facial expressions typical of adult grief, Darwin concluded (1872), are a resultant, on the one hand, of a tendency to scream like a child when he feels abandoned and, on the other, of an inhibition of such screaming. Both crying and screaming are, of course, ways by means of which a child commonly attracts and recovers his missing mother, or some other person who may help him find her; and they occur in grief, we believe, with the same objectives in mind – either consciously or unconsciously.

The frequency with which anger occurs as part of normal mourning has, we believe, habitually been underestimated – perhaps because it seems so out of place and shameful. Yet there can be no doubt about its very frequent occurrence especially in the early days. Both Lindemann and Marris were struck by it. It was evident, at least episodically, in eighteen out of the twenty-two widows studied by Parkes, and in seven of them it was very marked at the time of the first interview. Targets of this anger were a relative (four cases), clergy, doctors, or officials (five), and in four cases the dead husband himself. In most such cases the reason given for the anger was that the person in question was held either to have been in some part responsible for the death or to have been negligent in connection with it, either towards the dead man or to the widow.

Among the four widows who expressed anger towards their dead husband was one who burst out angrily during an interview nine months after her loss: 'Oh Fred, why did you leave me? If you had known what it was like, you'd never have left me'. Later, she denied she was angry and remarked, 'It's wicked to be angry'. Another widow also expressed angry reproach against her husband for his having deserted her.

Some degree of self-reproach was also common, and usually centred on some minor act of omission or commission associated with the last illness or the death. Although there were times when this self-reproach was fairly severe, in none of this series of widows was it as intense and unrelenting as it is in subjects whose grief persists until finally it becomes diagnosed as a depressive illness (Parkes 1965).

In the earlier paper (Bowlby 1961b), it was pointed out that anger is both usual and useful when separation is only temporary: it then helps overcome obstacles to reunion with the lost figure; and, after reunion is achieved, the expressions of reproach towards whoever seemed responsible for the separation make it less likely that a separation will occur again. Only when separation is permanent is the anger and reproach out of place.

It was concluded; there are therefore good biological reasons for every separation to be responded to in an automatic instinctive way with aggressive behaviour: irretrievable loss is statistically so unusual that it is not taken into account. In the course of our evolution, it appears, our instinctual equipment has come to be so fashioned that all losses are assumed to be retrievable and are responded to accordingly.

(Bowlby 1961b)

The hypothesis that many of the features of the second phase of mourning are to be understood as aspects not only of yearning but of actual searching for the lost figure is central to our whole thesis. It is intimately linked, of course, to the picture of attachment behaviour that one of us has advanced (Bowlby 1969). Attachment behaviour, it is argued, is a form of instinctive behaviour that develops in humans, as in other mammals, during infancy, and has as its aim or goal proximity to a mother-figure. The function of attachment behaviour, it is suggested, is protection from predators. Whilst attachment behaviour is shown especially strongly[1] during childhood when it is directed towards parent figures, it none the less continues to be active during adult life when it is usually directed towards some active and dominant figure, often a relative but sometimes an employer or some elder of the community. Attachment behaviour, the theory emphasizes, is elicited whenever a person (child or adult) is sick or in trouble, and is elicited at high intensity when he is frightened or when the attachment figure cannot be found. Because, in the light of this theory, attachment behaviour is regarded as a normal and healthy part of man's instinctive makeup, it is held to be most misleading to term it 'regressive' or childish when seen in older child or adult. For this reason, too, the term 'dependency' is regarded as leading to a seriously mistaken perspective: for in everyday speech to describe someone as dependent cannot help carrying with it overtones of criticism. By contrast, to describe someone as attached carries with it a positive evaluation.

This picture of attachment behaviour as a normal and healthy component of man's instinctive equipment leads us also to regard separation anxiety as the natural and inevitable response whenever an attachment figure is unaccountably missing. It is in the light of this hypothesis, we believe, that the panic attacks to which bereaved people are known to be prone can best be understood. They are apt to come on during the early months of bereavement, especially when the reality of loss happens to have been brought home to the bereaved.

Both our own small-scale but intensive study and also a larger survey reported by Maddison and Walker (1967) suggest that most women take a long time to get over the loss of a husband. By whatever psychiatric standard they are judged, less than a half are themselves again at the end of the first year. Of the twenty-two widows interviewed by Parkes, two were judged still to be grieving a great deal and nine more were intermittently disturbed and depressed. Only four seemed by the end of the first year to be making a good adjustment. Insomnia and a variety of minor aches and ailments were extremely common. In the survey undertaken by Maddison and Walker, one-fifth of the widows were still in very poor health and disturbed emotional state at the end of a year.

We emphasize these findings, distressing though they are, because we believe that clinicians sometimes have unrealistic expectations of the speed with which someone should get over a major bereavement. It is possible that some of Freud's theoretical formulations may have been a little misleading in this regard. For example, an oft-quoted passage from *Totem and Taboo* (1902–13) runs thus: 'Mourning has a quite precise psychical task to perform: its function is to detach the survivor's memories and hopes from the dead'. When judged by this criterion, it must be recognized, most mourning is unsuccessful. Freud himself was alive to this, however. Thus, in a letter of condolence to Binswanger (see E. L. Freud 1961), he writes:

Although we know that after such a loss the acute state of

> mourning will subside, we also know we shall remain inconsolable and will never find a substitute. No matter what may fill the gap, even if it be filled completely, it nevertheless remains something else. And actually this is how it should be. It is the only way of perpetuating that love which we do not want to relinquish.

The widows interviewed by Parkes a year after bereavement echoed these words. Over half of them still found it hard to accept the fact that their husband was dead: most of them still spent much time thinking about the past and still sometimes had a sense of their husband's nearby presence. In none of these widows had memories and hopes become detached from the dead.

In our own studies and also in those of Maddison and Walker it has been found that the younger a woman is when widowed the more intense her mourning and the more disturbed is her health likely to be at the end of twelve months. By contrast, if a woman is already over sixty-five when her husband dies, the blow is likely to be much less disabling. It seems as though the ties are already beginning to loosen. This quite marked difference in the intensity and length of mourning may perhaps provide a clue to understanding what happens following a loss during childhood.

GRIEF AND MOURNING IN CHILDHOOD

Some years ago one of us (Bowlby 1960b) emphasized that young children not only grieve but that they often do so for much longer than was sometimes supposed. In support of that view he quoted some of the observations of his colleagues – Robertson (1953b) and Heinicke (1956)* – of the persistent

* See also a later study by Heinicke and Westheimer (1966).

grieving for mother of one- and two-year-old children in residential nurseries, and also accounts of children in the Hampstead Nurseries during the war. These studies seem to make it clear that in those circumstances very young children grieve overtly for a missing mother for at least some weeks, crying for her or indicating in other ways that they are still yearning for her and expecting her return. The notion that grief in infancy and early childhood is short-lived does not bear scrutiny in the light of these observations. In particular the account given by Freud and Burlingham (1943) was cited of a boy aged three years and two months whose grief clearly persisted for some time though in muted form. We repeat that account now because we believe it contains so much of relevance. On being left in the nursery Patrick had been admonished to be a good boy and not to cry – otherwise his mother would not visit him.

Patrick tried to keep his promise and was not seen crying. Instead he would nod his head whenever anyone looked at him and assured himself and anybody who cared to listen that his mother would come for him, she would put on his overcoat and would take him home with her again. Whenever a listener seemed to believe him he was satisfied; whenever anybody contradicted him, he would burst into violent tears.

This same state of affairs continued through the next two or three days with several additions. The nodding took on a more compulsive and automatic character: My mother will put on my overcoat and take me home again.

Later an ever-growing list of clothes that his mother was supposed to put on him was added: She will put on my overcoat and my leggings, she will zip up the zipper, she will put on my pixie hat.

When the repetitions of this formula became monotonous and endless, somebody asked him whether he could not stop saying it all over again. Again Patrick tried to be the good boy that his mother wanted him to be. He stopped repeating the formula aloud, but his moving lips showed that he was saying it over and over to himself.

At the same time he substituted for the spoken words gestures that showed the position of his pixie hat, the putting on of an imaginary coat, the zipping of the zipper, etc. What showed as an expressive movement one day, was reduced the next to a mere abortive flicker of his fingers. While the other children were mostly busy with their toys, playing games, making music, etc., Patrick, totally uninterested, would stand somewhere in a corner, moving his hands and lips with an absolutely tragic expression on his face.

(Freud and Burlingham 1942: 89)

A good deal of controversy followed Bowlby's early papers; and we suspect it will be some time yet before all the problems raised are clarified. Of the many issues debated there are only two that we want to comment on here. The first concerns the usage of the term mourning; the second concerns the similarities and differences between childhood mourning and adult mourning.

In the earlier papers it was thought useful to use the term 'mourning' in a broad sense to cover a variety of reactions to loss, including some that lead to a pathological outcome and also those that follow loss in early childhood. The advantage of this usage is that it then becomes possible to link together a number of processes and conditions that evidence shows are interrelated – much in the way that the term 'inflammation' is used in physiology and pathology to link together a number of processes, some of which lead to a healthy outcome and some of which miscarry and result in pathology. The alternative practice is to restrict the term mourning to a particular form of reaction to loss, namely the one 'in which the lost object is gradually decathected by the painful and prolonged work of remembering and reality testing' (Wolfenstein 1966). A danger of that usage, however, is that it may lead to expectations of what healthy mourning should be like that are wholly at variance with what we now know actually occurs in many people. Furthermore, if the convention of a restricted usage is preferred, we find ourselves faced with the necessity of finding, and perhaps coining, some new term; for we believe it essential, if we are to discuss these matters productively, that we have some convenient word by which to refer to the whole range of processes that are brought into action when a loss is sustained. On this occasion we shall use the term 'grieving' in this sense, since it has already been employed by prominent analysts in a rather broad way and there is no dispute that very young children grieve.

In addition to having concentrated attention on a central area of psychopathology, the controversies of recent years have had a number of other effects that must be welcome to everyone. They have shown how little we yet know about how children of all ages, including adolescents, respond to a major loss and about what factors are responsible for outcome being more favourable in some cases than in others[2]; second, they have stimulated valuable research.

We have already emphasized how very difficult it is even for grown-ups to grasp fully that someone near to them is dead and will not return. For children it is clearly much more difficult still. Wolfenstein (1966) has reported on the responses of a number of children and adolescents who had lost a parent and who had come into analysis, many of them within a year of the bereavement. Amongst points that struck her group of observers was that 'sad feelings were curtailed; there was little weeping. Immersion in the activities of everyday life continued . . .' Yet gradually the analysts treating them became aware that overtly or covertly these children and adolescents were 'denying the finality of the loss' and that expectation that the lost parent would return was still present at a more or less conscious level.

The same long-persisting expectations are recorded by Barnes (1964) as occurring in two nursery school children who lost their mother when they were aged two-and-a-half and four years respectively. Again and again these children continued to express the hope and expectation that mother would return.

When in due course, through the help of analysts or others, these children gradually became aware that mother would, in fact, not return, they responded, as did the widows described above, with panic and anger. Ruth, a fifteen-year-old described by Wolfenstein, remarked some months after her mother had died, 'If my mother were really dead, I would be all alone . . . I would be terribly scared'. At another time it is recounted how Ruth, in bed at night, would sometimes feel desperate with 'frustration, rage and yearning. She tore the bedclothes off the bed, rolled them into the shape of a human body, and embraced them.'

Thus, although there certainly are differences between the way a child responds to loss and the way an adult does, there are also very basic similarities.

There is, moreover, one further similarity to which we wish to draw attention. Not only child but adult also, we believe, needs the assistance of another trusted person if he is to recover from the loss. In discussing the responses of children to loss, and how best to help them, almost every writer has emphasized how immensely important it is that a child have available a single and permanent substitute to whom he can gradually become attached. Only in such circumstances can we expect a child ultimately to accept the loss as irremediable and then to reorganize his inner life accordingly.* The same is true, we suspect, for

---

* How unsatisfactory any other arrangement is was poignantly expressed by Wendy, the four-year-old described by Barnes (1964). When her father enumerated the long list of people who knew Wendy and loved her, Wendy replied sadly, 'But when my Mummy wasn't dead I didn't need so many people – I needed just one.'

adults, although in adult life it may be a little easier to find support in the companionship of a few others as well. This leads to two interrelated and very practical questions: What do we know of the factors that aid or hinder healthy mourning? How can we best help a mourner?

CONDITIONS THAT AID OR HINDER HEALTHY MOURNING

It is now generally agreed amongst psychiatrists that, if mourning is to lead to a more rather than a less favourable outcome, it is necessary for a bereaved person – sooner or later – to express his feelings. 'Give sorrow words,' wrote Shakespeare, 'the grief that does not speak knits up the o'erwrought heart and bids it break.'

Yet, though so far we can all agree, for someone unable to express his feelings and for someone else trying to help him do so, the questions remain: how give sorrow words? what are the feelings to be expressed? and what is stopping their expression?

There is now evidence that the most intense and most disturbing affects aroused by loss are fear of being abandoned, yearning for the lost figure, and anger that he cannot be found – affects linked, on the one hand, with an urge to search for the lost figure and, on the other, with a tendency to reproach angrily anyone who seems to the bereaved to be responsible for the loss or to be hindering recovery of the lost person. With his whole emotional being, it seems, a bereaved person is fighting fate, trying desperately to turn back the wheel of time and to recapture the happier days that have been suddenly taken from him. So far from facing reality and trying to come to terms with it, a bereaved person is locked in a struggle with the past.

Plainly, if we are to give the kind of help to a bereaved person that we should all like to give, it is essential we see things from his point of view and respect his feelings – unrealistic though we may regard some of them to be. For only if a bereaved person feels we can at least understand and sympathize with him in the tasks he sets himself is there much likelihood that he will be able to express the feelings that are bursting within him – his yearning for the return of the lost figure, his hope against hope that miraculously all may yet be well, his rage at being deserted, his angry, unfair reproaches against 'those incompetent doctors', 'those unhelpful nurses', and against his own guilty self; if only he had done so and so, or not done so and so, disaster might perhaps have been averted.

Whether we are in the role of friend to a recently bereaved person or of therapist to someone who has suffered a bereavement many years ago and has failed in his mourning, it seems to be both unnecessary and unhelpful to cast ourselves in the role of a 'representative of reality': unnecessary because the bereaved is, in some part of himself, well aware that the world has changed; unhelpful because, by disregarding the world as one part of him still sees it, we alienate ourselves from him. Instead, our role should be that of companion and supporter, prepared to explore in our discussions all the hopes and wishes and dim unlikely possibilities that he still cherishes, together with all the regrets and the reproaches and the disappointments that afflict him. Let us give two examples.

In an earlier paper (Bowlby 1963), the case was described of Mrs. Q, a woman of about thirty-five; her father had died unexpectedly following an elective operation, and at a time when her therapist (J.B.) was abroad. For a year she had kept her feelings and her ideas to herself, but on the anniversary of the loss the true picture came out.

> During the weeks following her father's death, she now told me, she had lived in the half-held conviction that the hospital had made a mistake in identity and that any day they would 'phone to say he was alive and ready to return home. Furthermore, she

had felt specially angry with me because of a belief that, had I been available, I would have been able to exert an influence on the hospital and so enable her to recover him. Now, twelve months later, these ideas and feelings persisted. She was still half-expecting a message from the hospital, and she was still angry with me for not approaching the authorities there. Secretly, moreover, she was still making arrangements to greet her father on his return. This explained why she had been so angry with her mother for redecorating the flat in which the old people had lived together and why too she had continued to postpone having her own flat redecorated: it was vital, she felt, that when at last her father did return he should find the places familiar.

(Bowlby 1963)

Now there was no need for her therapist to intervene on behalf of reality: others had already done so and she knew well enough what view of the world was held by her relatives and friends. What she needed was the chance to express the yearning, the hopes, and the bitter anger that her relatives and friends could not understand. She described how the previous week she had thought she had seen her father looking into a shop window and how she had crossed the road to inspect more closely the man in question. She described her fury with the staff nurse who had given her the news of her father's death and how she had felt inclined to throw her on the concrete floor and bash her brains out. She described how she felt her therapist had failed her by being away just when she most wanted him; and she described much else besides that, in the cold light of day, she herself knew was unrealistic and unfair. What she needed from the therapist, and we hope found, was someone who could understand and sympathize with her unrealism and her unfairness. As the months rolled by, her hopes and her anger faded and she began to reconcile herself to the reality of loss.

The same role was played with a boy of sixteen, whom we shall call Bill. He had first been seen by a psychiatrist (J.B.) at a clinic when he was four years old because things were going badly in his foster home. The history was uncertain but we gathered that Bill's mother was a prostitute who had placed her son in a foster home when he was two years old and had then disappeared. Bill presented great problems and the foster parents refused to keep him. Special foster care was arranged and, later, treatment in a residential establishment for seriously disturbed children. A few times a year he was seen at the clinic by the same psychiatrist and in that way we provided some continuity. Now at sixteen he was due to leave school soon.

In that interview Bill told the psychiatrist of his plan to go to America to find his mother. He had already been to a steamship company and was arranging to work his passage over. He was quite an intelligent boy and his plans for transport seemed practicable. Yet you can imagine the psychiatrist's astonishment! Here was a boy who had last seen his mother when he was two and had never heard from her since, who had no idea where she might be, and who was not even sure of her name. Plainly the scheme was a wild goose chase. Yet, the psychiatrist held his tongue. This was Bill's world and Bill's plan, and he was confiding it to his therapist; it was not the latter's role to debunk it. In fact a whole session was spent discussing the plan. Bill believed his father was an American serviceman and he presumed his mother had returned with him after the war. His plans for crossing the Atlantic were looked at again and the methods whereby he might earn enough on the other side to continue his search. No queries were raised by the psychiatrist, but Bill was invited to come back for a further talk in a week or so. He came back. He described how he had been thinking a great deal about the plan but was beginning to have doubts. Perhaps it would be difficult to locate his mother; and perhaps, even if he were successful, she might not be too welcoming. After all, he reflected, he would be a stranger to her. Once again, given a chance to explore in sympathetic company all the feelings and plans that he had nursed secretly for years, the patient's own sense of reality was sufficient.

Naturally in other patients, especially older ones who have suffered a loss years earlier during childhood or adolescence, to help them recover their lost feelings, their lost hopes of reunion, and their anger at being deserted, can be a long and technically difficult task. But the overall aims remain the same.

Yearning for the impossible, intemperate anger, impotent weeping, horror at the prospect of loneliness, pitiful pleading for sympathy and support – these are the feelings that a bereaved person needs to express, and sometimes first to discover, if he is to make progress. Yet, these are all feelings that are apt to be regarded as unworthy and unmanly. At best to express them may seem humiliating; at worst it may be to court criticism and contempt. No wonder such feelings so often go unexpressed, and may later go underground.

This leads us to the question why some people find it harder – often much harder – to express their feelings of grief than do others.

Our own belief is that a main reason why some find expressing grief extremely difficult is that the family in which they have been brought up, and with which they still mix, is one in which the attachment behaviour of a child is regarded unsympathetically as something to be grown out of as quickly as possible. In such families crying and other protests over separation are apt to be dubbed babyish, and anger or jealousy as reprehensible. In such families, moreover, the more a child demands to be with his mother or his father the more he is told that such demands are silly and unjustified; the more he cries or throws a tantrum the more he is told he is babyish and bad. As a result of being subjected to such pressures he is likely to come to accept these standards for himself; to cry, to make demands, to feel angry because they are not met, to blame others, will all be judged by him as unjustified, babyish, and bad. So, when he suffers serious loss, instead of expressing the kinds of feelings that every bereaved person is filled with, he is inclined to stifle them. Furthermore, his relatives, products of the same family culture, are likely to share the same critical outlook towards emotion and its expression. And so the very person who most needs understanding and encouragement is the one least likely to receive it.

A vivid illustration of this process of internalization of reproachful controls is provided by the case of Patrick, the three-year-old boy in the Hampstead Nursery described earlier. Patrick, you will remember, had been admonished to be a good boy and not to cry – otherwise his mother would not visit him. It seems likely that this was typical of her attitude towards his expressions of distress. It is therefore not surprising that he strove to stifle all his feelings and, instead of expressing them, developed a ritual that became increasingly divorced from the emotional context in which it had originated.

Avoidance of mourning is one important pathological variant of grief but it is not, we believe, the only one. There are many bereaved adults seeking help from psychiatrists who show little evidence of the inhibition of emotion that has been described above. On the contrary, as is documented in a previous paper (Parkes 1965), these people are showing all the features of grief in a severe and protracted form. The problem here is not one of why the patient is unable to express grief but why she (and it is usually a woman) is unable to get over it. It may be, of course, that even in these cases there is some as yet unrecognized component of grief that is being inhibited; but there are three characteristics which seem to distinguish these chronic grief reactions and which may suggest an alternative explanation.

In the first place the patient's attachment to her lost spouse is usually found to have been an extremely close one, with a great deal of the self-esteem and role identity of the survivor dependent on the continued presence of the spouse. Such patients are likely to report having experienced great distress even during brief temporary separations in the past. Second, the patient has no close relationship with another family member towards whom she can transfer some of the ties which bound her to her husband. Her intense relationship with him seems to have been so exclusive that even those family members who exist have drifted away, so that after bereavement the survivor has found no person and no interests to distract her from her grief. Finally, the marriage relationship is likely to have been an ambivalent one, perhaps because the husband resented the possessiveness of his wife. At all events the survivor usually finds some source of self-reproach and castigates herself for having failed to be a better wife or for having allowed her husband to die. The grief of such people often seems to contain an element of self-punishment, as if perpetual mourning had become a sacred duty to the dead by means of which the survivor could make retribution.

The treatment of such patients is likely to prove difficult as they often seem to relish the opportunity to repeat, yet again, the painful drama of their loss. While there is no general agreement as to the value of psychotherapy for them, much can be done to help re-establish their commitment to the world. Family, local clergy, or the befriending service of an organization such as Cruse or Samaritans, can be mobilized to act as a bridge; whilst a memorial service, a holiday with friends, or even the redecoration of the home can be a turning point, a *rite-de-passage*, out of the role of mourner to the new role of widow.

Seen in this light, bereavement becomes a family problem. Therefore, we need to know what changes occur in the dynamic structure of a family when a leading member dies. Relevant information is emerging from a study of young Boston widows and widowers currently in progress.[3] Apart from emotional problems the most immediate problem is one of roles. Who, for example, is to take over the roles of a dead husband? Some of them, such as the management of household affairs, commonly devolve upon the surviving widow. Others remain unfilled: thus many widows sleep with a pillow or bolster in bed beside them. A young widow will usually try to perceive her dead husband as a continuing help in decision making, and to make his wishes and preferences the ground for much of her own behaviour. When decisions must be made that fall outside the field of this 'internal referee', she will most often turn to her husband's brother as the person closest to the husband in culture and blood. Similarly, a widower tends to regard his sister-in-law as the most helpful member of his wife's family and to seek her help in making decisions about children and household affairs.

As time passes, however, these role assignments fade and are followed often by a gradual disintegration of the extended family. The widow or widower no longer looks to the spouse's family as a source of support and, instead, develops a greater degree of self-reliance, despite the loneliness and internal family strains that this entails. Friends and children then become an important source of affirmation as the widow or widower develops a tougher stance and tackles the world afresh.

The ability of a widow or widower to cope with these fresh roles and responsibilities clearly depends partly on personality and previous experience and partly on the demands made by and the support found in the family environment. Children may be a burden or a blessing, so may in-laws; and the woman without experience of a job outside the home has many hurdles to negotiate. It is not surprising that a significant proportion of widows fail to find any satisfying mode of living. When asked thirteen months after bereavement how they felt, 74 per cent of the young Boston widows agreed that 'you never get over it'.

A study that illustrates the part that friends and relatives play in influencing the outcome of bereavement has been carried out by Maddison and Walker (1967). They studied two groups of widows, each of twenty subjects who had agreed to be interviewed, and matched as far as possible on the usual sociological variables. One group had been selected because at the end of twelve months they all seemed, on the basis of their health records, to have reached a fairly favourable outcome; the other group were selected because their health records suggested that outcome had not been favourable. Interviews confirmed that the health record is in fact a good index of how a person is coping with the emotional problems of bereavement.

During the course of long semi-structured interviews, the interviewer inquired who had been available to the window during her first three months of widowhood, and in regard to each whether she had found them helpful, unhelpful, or neutral. In addition, questions were directed to finding out whether the widow had found it easy or difficult to express her feelings with each person mentioned, whether or not they had encouraged her to dwell on the past, whether they had been eager to direct her attention to problems of the present and future, and whether they had offered practical help. Since the object of the inquiry was to find out only how the widows themselves recalled their dealings with others, no attempt was made to check how their accounts may have tallied with those of the people with whom they had been in contact.

When the replies of the two groups of widows were compared, the following differences stood out. First, widows whose condition after twelve months was unfavourable reported that they had received too little encouragement either to express their grief and anger, or to talk about their dead husband and the past. They complained that, instead, people seemed to have made expression of feeling more difficult by insisting that she pull herself together or control herself, that anyway she was not the only one to suffer, that she would be wise to face the problems of the future rather than dwell unproductively on the past. By contrast, widows with a fairly good outcome reported how the people they had been in contact with had made it easy for them to cry and to express the intensity of their feelings; and they described what a relief it had been to be able to talk freely and at length about past days with their husband and the circumstances of his death.

How are we to interpret these findings? An obvious explanation, and perhaps the most likely, is that the attitude of these friends and relatives caused the widow to suppress or avoid expression of grief and that the pathological outcome had occurred as a consequence of this. Alternatively, the widow may have attributed to her friends and relatives her own fear of expressing feeling and blamed them for her own incapacity. Or both processes may have occurred together.

Yet the forms of pathological outcome described by Maddison and Walker are not all attributable to inhibition or avoidance of grief; there were several widows who showed the chronic grief syndrome described above. In these cases it is possible that the experiences the widows reported reflect a breakdown in communication such that the family were not seen as sympathetic and helpful. Lacking their understanding and support, the widow may well have found it difficult to find any inducement to start again, to commit herself to a new investment in the world with all the dangers of further disappointment and loss. Instead, it seems she had tended to look backwards, to search repeatedly for the husband she could find only in memory, and to condemn herself to persistent grief.

This brings us to our final point. We are uneasy about some of the theory that is presented in the psychoanalytic literature and about some of the language that is used in clinical discussion. For example, it is not unusual to find the weeping of grown-ups after a disastrous loss referred to as 'a regression' or the strong longing for the company of another person, an urge to cling, described as being the expression of 'infantile dependence'. Not only do we believe such theorizing to be mistaken on scientific grounds but it plainly represents an attitude which, if carried over to clinical work, can only reinforce the tendencies of a bereaved person to feel guilty and ashamed of the very feelings and behaviour we believe it will help him most to express.

There are other words and concepts that we believe lead to the same difficulties. 'Magical thinking' and 'fantasy' are terms to be used with extreme caution. A fantasy is by definition something wholly unrealistic; so that to refer to a child's hopes and expectations of her dead mother's return as a 'wishful fantasy' is, in our eyes, to do them less than justice. Mrs. Q's belief that her father might still be alive was, we believe, likely to be mistaken as she herself suspected, but it was not absurd. Mistakes are made occasionally, and missing people do return when least expected. The ideas of Bill, the sixteen-year-old boy who hoped to find his mother, were probably misconceived but given certain premises it was a legitimate enough plan. By avoiding such loaded terms as 'denial of reality' and 'fantasy' and using, instead, phrases such as 'disbelief that X has occurred', 'belief that Y may still be possible', or 'making a plan to achieve Z', it seems to us that we are able to see the world more as our patients see it and to maintain that neutral and empathic position from which, we know from experience, we are best able to help them.

NOTES

1   See note 1 to Chapter 3.
2   Much more is now known about the conditions that affect the course of childhood mourning. See notes 4 and 5 to Chapter 3.
3   See the book by Glick, Weiss, and Parkes (1974).

6

SELF-RELIANCE AND SOME CONDITIONS THAT PROMOTE IT*

In the autumn of 1970 the Tavistock Clinic celebrated the Golden Jubilee of its foundation. To mark the event the Clinic and its sister organization, the Tavistock Institute of Human Relations, organized a conference at which papers describing work going forward in the two institutions were presented. A version of this paper was included, and an amplified version published later in the proceedings of the conference.

THE CONCEPT OF SECURE BASE

Evidence is accumulating that human beings of all ages are happiest and able to deploy their talents to best advantage when

* Originally published in Gosling, R. G. (ed.) (1973) *Support, Innovation and Autonomy*. London: Tavistock Publications. Reprinted by permission of The Tavistock Institute of Human Relations.

they are confident that, standing behind them, there are one or more trusted persons who will come to their aid should difficulties arise. The person trusted, also known as an attachment figure (Bowlby 1969), can be considered as providing his (or her) companion with a secure base from which to operate.

The requirement of an attachment figure, a secure personal base, is by no means confined to children though, because of its urgency during the early years, it is during those years that it is most evident and has been most studied. There are good reasons for believing, however, that the requirement applies also to adolescents and to mature adults as well. In the latter, admittedly, the requirement is commonly less evident, and it probably differs both between the sexes and at different phases of life. For those reasons and also for reasons stemming from the values of western culture, the requirement of adults for a secure base tends often to be overlooked, or even denigrated.

In the picture of personality functioning that emerges there are two main sets of influences. The first concerns the presence or absence, partial or total, of a trustworthy figure willing and able to provide the kind of secure base required at each phase of the life-cycle. These constitute the external, or environmental, influences. The second set concerns the relative ability or inability of an individual, first, to recognize when another person is both trustworthy and willing to provide a base and, second, when recognized, to collaborate with that person in such a way that a mutually rewarding relationship is initiated and maintained. These constitute the internal, or organismic, influences.

Throughout life the two sets of influences interact in complex and circular ways. In one direction the kinds of experience a person has, especially during childhood, greatly affect both whether he expects later to find a secure personal base, or not, and also the degree of competence he has to initiate and maintain a mutually rewarding relationship when opportunity offers. In the reverse direction the nature of the expectations a person has, and the degree of competence he brings, play a large part in determining both the kinds of person with whom he associates and how they then treat him. Because of these interactions, whatever pattern is first established tends to persist. This is a main reason why the pattern of family relationships a person experiences during childhood is of such crucial importance for the development of his personality.

Looked at in this light healthy personality functioning at every age reflects, first, an individual's ability to recognize suitable figures willing and able to provide him with a secure base and, second, his ability to collaborate with such figures in mutually rewarding relationships. By contrast, many forms of disturbed personality functioning reflect an individual's imparied ability to recognize suitable and willing figures and/or an impaired ability to collaborate in rewarding relationships with any such figure when found. Such impairment can be of every degree and take many forms: they include anxious clinging, demands excessive or over-intense for age and situation, aloof non-committal, and defiant independence.

Paradoxically, the healthy personality when viewed in this light proves by no means as independent as cultural stereotypes suppose. Essential ingredients are a capacity to rely trustingly on others when occasion demands and to know on whom it is appropriate to rely. A healthily functioning person is thus capable of exchanging roles when the situation changes. At one time he is providing a secure base from which his companion or companions can operate; at another he is glad to rely on one or another of his companions to provide him with just such a base in return.

A capacity to adopt either role as circumstances change is well-illustrated by many women during successive phases of their lives running from pregnancy through childbirth and on into motherhood. A woman capable of coping successfully with these shifts is found by Wenner (1966) well able, during her pregnancy and puerperium, both to express her desire for support and help and also to do so in a direct and effective fashion to an appropriate figure. Her relationship with her husband is close and she is eager and content to rely on his support. In her turn she is able to give spontaneously to others, including her baby. By contrast, Wenner reports, a woman who experiences major emotional difficulties during pregnancy and puerperium is found to have great difficulty in relying on others. She is either unable to express her desire for support or else she does so in a demanding aggressive way, in either case reflecting her lack of confidence that it will be forthcoming. Commonly she is both dissatisfied with what she may be given and is herself unable to give spontaneously to others.

In order to provide the continuity of potential support that is the essence of a secure base, the relationships between the individuals concerned must persist over a period of time, measured in terms of years. Although, for clarity of exposition, theory is often best formulated in non-feeling terms, it must be borne constantly in mind that many of the most intense human emotions arise during the formation, the maintenance, the disruption, and the renewal of those relationships in which one partner is providing a secure base for the other, or in which they alternate roles. Whereas the unchallenged maintenance of such relationships is experienced as a source of security, threat of loss gives rise to anxiety and often to anger, and actual loss to the turmoil of feeling that is grief.

The theoretical position proposed includes a number of concepts familiar in psychoanalytic object relations theory; for example, Fairbairn's concept of mature dependency and Winnicott's concept of the facilitating environment (Fairbairn 1952; Winnicott 1965). It differs, however, from traditional clinical theory at a number of points. One is the avoidance of the terms 'dependence' and 'dependency needs', which, it is held, are in part responsible for very serious confusion in existing theory. A second is to attribute importance for development to experiences during all the years of childhood and adolescence instead of almost exclusively to the earliest months or years. Others are that the schema proposed is cast in terms of control theory and that it draws not only on clinical data but also on the findings of a broad range of descriptive and experimental studies both of humans and of non-human primates.*

The aims of this paper are to indicate some of the evidence that supports the viewpoint sketched, to consider briefly what is known of the conditions that favour or impede the development of healthy personality as here conceived, and, if possible, to clarify theoretical issues that have proved troublesome.

STUDIES OF SELF-RELIANT MEN AND YOUTHS

During the past decade or two a number of clinicians have turned their attention to the study of individuals who, it is reasonable to believe, possess well-functioning and healthy personalities. Not only do these people show none of the usual signs of personality disturbance, either in the present or, as far as can be told, in their past, but they are plainly self-reliant and successful both in their human relationships and their work. Though each of the studies so far published is inadequate in a number of ways, findings are suggestive. First, these well-adapted personalities show a smoothly working balance of, on the one hand, initiative and self-reliance, and, on the other, a capacity both to seek help and to make use of help when occasion demands. Second, an examination of their development shows that they have grown up in closely knit families with parents who, it

---

* Both the theory itself and the evidence on which it rests are presented at greater length in the first and second volumes of *Attachment and Loss* (Bowlby 1969 and 1973).

seems, have never failed to provide them with support and encouragement. Third, though here evidence is less substantial, the family itself has been and still is part of a stable social network within which a growing child is welcome and can mix both with other adults and with peers, many of whom are familiar to him from his earliest years.

So far as it goes, each study gives the same picture, the picture of a stable family base from which first the child, then the adolescent and finally the young adult moves out in a series of ever-lengthening excursions. Whilst autonomy is evidently encouraged in such families, it is not forced. Each step follows the previous one in a series of easy stages. Though home ties may be attenuated they are never broken.

Astronauts rank high as self-reliant men capable of living and working effectively in conditions of great potential danger and stress. Their performance, their personalities, and their histories have been studied by Korchin and Ruff. In two articles (Korchin and Ruff 1964; Ruff and Korchin 1967) they publish preliminary findings on a small sample of seven men.

Despite a high degree of self-reliance and a clear preference for independent action, all the men are reported to be 'comfortable when dependence on others is required' and to have a 'capacity to maintain trust, in what might seem conditions of distrust'. The performance of the crew of Apollo 13, which met with a mishap en route to the moon, is testimony to their capacity in this respect. Not only did they maintain their own efficiency in conditions of great danger but they continued to cooperate trustingly and effectively with their companions at the base on earth.

Turning to their life histories we find that these men 'grew up in relatively small well-organized communities, with considerable family solidarity and strong identification with the father . . . [They showed] a relatively smooth growth pattern in which they could meet available challenges, increase levels of aspiration, succeed and gain further confidence, and in this way grow in competence'.

Another study, this time of young men at college who appeared to their teachers to be of good general mental health and to promise well as youth leaders and community workers, is reported by Grinker (1962).

Among the sixty-five students interviewed Grinker regarded only a handful as showing neurotic character structure. The large majority seemed straightforward youths, honest and accurate in their self-evaluations, with a 'capacity for close and deep human relationships . . . to members of their families, peers, teachers and to the interviewer'. Their reports of experiencing anxiety or sadness suggested that such feelings arose in appropriate situations and were neither severe nor prolonged.

As regards their experience of home life, the overall picture reported by the students is remarkably similar to that reported by the astronauts. In almost every case both parents were still alive. The typical picture presented was of a happy peaceful home in which both parents shared responsibilities and interests, and were regarded by the children as loving and giving. During childhood, they said, they had felt with mother above everything else secure. At the same time they had identified strongly with father. Grinker reports much further evidence in support of these conclusions.

The findings both of a developmental study, from age ten to seventeen years, of thirty-four adolescents of very different characters (Peck and Havighurst 1960) and also of a small study of successful students during their transition from high school to first year in college (Murphey et al. 1963) are very similar to Grinker's. Evidence presented suggests that both self-reliance and the capacity to rely on others are alike products of a family that provides strong support for its offspring combined with respect for their personal aspirations, their sense of responsibility, and their ability to deal with the world. So far from sapping a child's self-reliance, it seems clear, strong family support can encourage it. Similar findings are reported from a more recent study of seventy-three teenage boys (Offer 1969).

This same pattern of self-reliance resting on a secure attachment to a trusted figure, and developing from it, can be seen as early as a child's first birthday. Whether these early patterns are true forerunners of later ones, or not, must await further research. To those with experience of family psychiatry, however, it seems probable that they are.

DEVELOPMENT DURING INFANCY

Since Freud's earliest work a main tenet of psychoanalysis has been that the foundations of personality are laid during the early years of childhood. Opinion has differed, however, as to which years are the most important, what psychological processes are involved and what experiences are influential in determining outcome. So long as relevant empirical data were lacking it was inevitable that debate should reach deadlock. Now, however, thanks to the work of psychoanalysts, clinically oriented psychologists and ethologists, the position is changing. Though data are still woefully insufficient, enough are available to permit an attempt at a systematic articulation of data and theory. Thanks to developments in theoretical biology, moreover, theory can itself be reformulated in ways better suited to the data. Thus prospects for advance are now good.

Amongst those in the van of this movement is Mary Salter Ainsworth who, since working at the Tavistock between 1950 and 1954, has continued to study problems of attachment and separation. Resulting from this she has published a naturalistic study of mother-infant interaction in Uganda (Ainsworth 1967) and is now presenting results of a planned study of mother-infant interaction in white middle-class homes in Baltimore, Maryland.

During her study of infancy in Uganda Ainsworth noticed how infants, once mobile, commonly use mother as a base from which to explore. When conditions are favourable they move away from mother on exploratory excursions and return to her again from time to time. By eight months of age almost every infant observed who had had a stable mother-figure to whom to become attached showed this behaviour; but should mother be absent such organized excursions became much less evident or ceased. Subsequently Anderson (1972) has made similar observations of exploration from a base of children aged between fifteen months and two and a half years playing in a secluded part of a London park whilst mother sits quietly on a seat.

In her carefully planned project in Baltimore, Ainsworth is not only able to study this kind of behaviour more closely but has described many individual variations of it to be seen in a sample of twenty-three infants* at twelve months of age. Observations have been made of the infants' exploratory and attachment behaviour, and the balance between them, both when the infants are at home with mother and also when they are placed in a slightly strange test situation. In addition, having obtained data on the type of mothering each infant had been receiving throughout his first year of life (by means of prolonged observation sessions at three-weekly intervals in the child's home), Ainsworth is in a position to propose hypotheses linking certain types of behavioural organization at twelve months with certain types of preceding mothering experience. The project is described and preliminary findings reported in Ainsworth and Bell (1970); individual differences and their antecedents are discussed in Ainsworth, Bell, and Stayton (1971, 1974).

The findings of the study show that, with only few exceptions,

* Although the total sample studied in the strange situation comprises fifty-six infants, only twenty-three of them have been observed also with mother at home.

the way a particular infant of twelve months behaves with and without his mother at home and the way he behaves with and without her in a slightly strange test situation have much in common. Drawing on observations of behaviour in both types of situation it is then possible to classify the infants into five main groups, according to two criteria: (a) how much or how little they explore when in different situations and (b) how they treat mother – when she is present, when she departs and when she returns.*

The five groups, with the number of infants classifiable into each, are as follows:

GROUP P: The exploratory behaviour of an infant in this group varies with the situation and is most evident in mother's presence. He uses mother as a base, keeps note of her whereabouts, and exchanges glances with her. From time to time he returns to her and enjoys contact with her. When she returns after a brief absence he greets her warmly. No ambivalence towards her is evident. N = 8.

GROUP Q: The behaviour of these infants is much like that of infants in Group P. Where it differs is, first, that infants in this group tend to explore more actively in the strange situation, and, second, they tend to be somewhat ambivalent towards mother.

* The classification presented here, based on behaviour in *both* types of situation, is a slightly modified version of one presented by Ainsworth *et al.* (1971) in which a child's behaviour in his own home is the *sole* source of data. Infants classified here into groups P, Q, and R are identical with the infants classified into Ainsworth's Groups I, II, and III. Those classified here into Group T are the same as those classified into Ainsworth's Group V, less one infant who, although passive at home, proved markedly independent in the strange situation test and is therefore transferred to Group S. The infants in Group S are the same as in Ainsworth's Group IV plus the one infant transferred. The classification presented here has Professor Salter Ainsworth's approval.

On the one hand, if ignored by her, an infant may become intensely demanding; on the other, he may ignore or avoid her in return. Yet at other times the pair are capable of happy exchanges together. N = 4.

GROUP R: An infant in this group explores very actively whether mother is present or absent, and whether the situation is familiar or strange. He tends, moreover, to have little to do with his mother, and is often not interested in being picked up by her. At other times, especially after his mother has left him alone in the strange situation, he behaves in a very contrary way, alternately seeking proximity to her and then avoiding it, or seeking contact and then wriggling away. N = 3.

GROUP S: The behaviour of infants in this group is inconsistent. Sometimes they appear very independent, though usually for brief periods only; at others they seem markedly anxious regarding mother's whereabouts. They are distinctly ambivalent about contact with her, seeking it frequently yet not seeming to enjoy it when given, or even strongly resisting it. Oddly enough, in the strange situation they tend to ignore mother's presence and to avoid both proximity and contact with her. N = 5.

GROUP T: These infants tend to be passive both at home and in the strange situation. They show relatively little exploratory behaviour but much auto-erotic behaviour. They are conspicuously anxious about mother's whereabouts and cry much in her absence; yet they can be markedly ambivalent to her when she returns. N = 3.

When an attempt is made to evaluate these different patterns of behaviour as forerunners of future personality development the eight children in Group S and T seem the least likely to develop a stable self-reliance combined with trust in others. Some are passive in both situations; others explore but only briefly.

Most of them seem anxious about mother's whereabouts, and relations with her tend to be extremely ambivalent.

The three children in Group R are most active in exploration and appear strongly independent. Yet their relations with mother are cautious, even slightly detached. To a clinician they give the impression of being unable to trust others, and to have developed a premature independence.

The four children in Group Q are more difficult to assess. They seem to lie half-way between those in Group R and those in Group P.

If the perspective adopted in this paper proves correct, it would be the eight children in Group P who would be most likely in due course to develop a stable self-reliance combined with trust in others; for they move freely and confidently between a busy interest in exploring their environment, and the people and things in it, and keeping in intimate touch with mother. It is true that they often show less self-reliance than those in Groups Q and R, and that in the strange situation they are more affected than the latter by mother's brief absences. Yet their relations with mother seem always to be cheerful and confident, whether expressed in affectionate embraces or in the exchanging of glances and vocalizations at a distance, and this seems to promise well for their future.

When the type of mothering received by each of these infants is examined, using data obtained during the long visits the observers paid to the home every three weeks during the infant's first year of life, interesting differences appear between infants in each of the five groups.

In assessing a mother's behaviour towards her child Ainsworth uses four distinct nine-point rating scales. Ratings on these scales intercorrelate so highly, however, that in this paper the results of only one scale are drawn upon. This is a scale that measures the degree of sensitivity or insensitivity that a mother shows to her baby's signals and communications. Whereas a sensitive mother seems constantly to be 'tuned in' to receive her baby's signals, is likely to interpret them correctly and to respond to them both promptly and appropriately, an insensitive mother will often not notice her baby's signals, will misinterpret them when she does notice them, and will then respond tardily, inappropriately, or not at all.

When the ratings on this scale for the mothers of infants in each of the five groups are examined, it is found that the mothers of the eight infants in Group P rate uniformly high (range 5.5 to 9.0), those of the eleven infants in Groups R, S, and T rate uniformly low (range 1.0 to 3.5), and those of the four in Group Q are in the middle (range 4.5 to 5.5). These differences are statistically significant (using the Mann-Whitney U test).

Differences between groups, in the same direction and of roughly the same order of magnitude, are found when mothers are rated on the other three scales. Thus mothers of infants in Group P are rated highly on an acceptance–rejection scale, a cooperation–interference scale and on an accessibility–ignoring scale. Conversely, mothers of infants in Groups R, S, and T are rated medium to low on each of these three scales. Mothers of infants in Group Q show ratings that lie roughly midway between the ratings for mothers of infants in Group P and those of infants in Groups R, S, and T respectively.

Plainly a very great deal of further work will be required before it is possible to draw conclusions with any high degree of confidence. Nevertheless the overall patterns of personality development and of mother–child interaction visible at twelve months are sufficiently similar to what is seen of personality development and of parent–child interaction in later years for it to be plausible to believe that the one is the forerunner of the other. At the least, Ainsworth's findings show that an infant whose mother is sensitive, accessible, and responsive to him, who accepts his behaviour and is cooperative in dealing with him, is far from being the demanding and unhappy child that some theories might suggest. Instead, mothering of this sort is evidently compatible with a child who is developing a limited measure of self-reliance by the time of his first birthday combined with a high degree of trust in his mother and enjoyment of her company.[1]

Further strong evidence pointing in this direction is presented by Baumrind (1967) who made a very detailed study of thirty-two nursery school children, aged three and four years, and their mothers.

Thus, so far as the present all too meagre evidence goes, the hypothesis that a well-found self-reliance develops in parallel with reliance on a parent, who provides the child with a secure base from which to explore, is sustained.

POINTS OF DIFFERENCE TO CURRENT THEORETICAL FORMULATIONS

Although the theoretical schema presented here is not very different from that adopted implicitly by many practising clinicians, it differs at a number of points from much currently taught theory. Among these differences are the following:

(a) An emphasis in the present schema on the environmental parameter familiar–strange, which finds no place in traditional theory;

(b) Emphasis in the present schema on the many components of mother–infant interaction other than feeding, an overemphasis on which, it is held, has greatly hindered our understanding of personality development and the conditions that influence it;

(c) The replacement of the concepts 'dependence' and 'independence' by the concepts of attachment, trust, reliance, and self-reliance;

(d) The replacement of the orally derived theory of internal objects by a theory of working models of world and self that are conceived as being constructed by each individual as a result of his experience, that determine his expectations, and on the basis of which he plans.

Let us consider in turn each of these differences, which are closely interrelated.

The immense importance in the lives of animals and men of the parameter familiar-strange has been fully recognized only during the past two decades, long after the various versions of clinical theory still taught had been formulated. In very many species, it is now known, whatever situation has become familiar to an individual is treated as though it provided safety, whereas any other situation is treated with reserve. Strangeness is responded to ambivalently; on the one hand it elicits fear and withdrawal, on the other it elicits curiosity and investigation. Which of these antithetic responses become dominant depends on many variables, the degree of strangeness of the situation, the presence or absence of a companion, and whether the individual responding is mature or immature, fit or fatigued, healthy or sick.

Why the properties of familiarity and strangeness should have come to have such powerful effects on behaviour is discussed in the final section of the paper, with special reference to their role in protection.

So long as the influence on man's behaviour of familiarity and strangeness was not appreciated, the conditions leading a child to become attached to his mother were little understood. The most plausible view, subscribed to by Freud and most other analysts and also by learning theorists, was that being fed by mother was the major variable. This theory, a theory of second-ary drive, although never supported by systematic evidence or argument, soon became widely accepted and led naturally to two other views both of which have attracted a strong following. One is that what happens during the early months of life must be of very special importance for later development. The second is that, once a child has learned to feed himself, there is no further reason for him to be demanding of his mother's presence: he should therefore grow out of such 'dependency', which is thence-forward stigmatized as infantile or babyish.

The view taken here, and supported by much evidence (Bowlby 1969), is that food plays only a marginal role in a child's attachment to his mother, that attachment behaviour is shown most strongly[2] during the second and third years of life and persists at less intensity indefinitely, and that the function of attachment behaviour is protection. Corollaries of this view are that involuntary separation and loss are potentially traumatic over many years of infancy, childhood, and adolescence, and that, at appropriate degrees of intensity, the propensity to show attachment behaviour is a healthy characteristic and in no sense infantile.

From out of the same traditional assumption, that a child becomes attached to his mother because of his dependence upon her as the source of his physiological gratifications, come the concepts and terminology of 'dependence' and 'independence'. Once a child can provide for himself, say advocates of the theory of secondary drive, he should become independent. Hence-forward, therefore, signs of dependency are to be regarded as regressive. Thus, once again, any strong desire for the presence of an attachment figure comes to be regarded as an expression of an 'infantile need', part of a 'baby' self that should have been left behind.

As terms and concepts in which to express the theory advanced here 'dependence' and 'independence' have a number of grave objections; they are therefore replaced by terms and concepts such as 'trust in', 'attached to', 'reliance on', and 'self-reliance'. First, dependence and independence are inevitably conceived as being mutually exclusive; whereas, as already emphasized, reliance on others and self-reliance are not only compatible but complementary to one another. Second, to describe someone as 'dependent' inevitably carries with it a pejorative flavour, whereas to describe someone as 'relying on another' does not. Third, whereas the concept of attachment implies always attachment to one (or more) specially loved person(s), the concept of dependency entails no such relationship but instead tends to be anonymous.

Also much influenced by the special role given to feeding and orality in psychoanalytic theorizing is the concept of 'internal object', a concept that is in many ways ambiguous (Strachey 1941). In its place can be put the concept, derived from cognitive psychology and control theory, of an individual developing within himself one or more working models representing principal features of the world about him and of himself as an agent in it. Such working models determine his expectations and forecasts and provide him with tools for constructing plans of action.

What in traditional theory is termed a 'good object' can be reformulated within this framework as a working model of an attachment figure who is conceived as accessible, trustworthy, and ready to help when called upon. Similarly, what in traditional theory is termed a 'bad object' can be reformulated as a working model of an attachment figure to whom are attributed such characteristics as uncertain accessibility, unwillingness to respond helpfully, or perhaps the likelihood of responding hostilely. In an analogous way an individual is thought to construct a working model of himself towards whom others will respond in certain predictable ways. The concept of a working model of the self comprehends data at present conceived in terms of self-image, self-esteem, etc.

The extent to which such working models are valid products of a child's actual experience over the years or are distorted versions of such experience is a matter of the greatest importance. Work in family psychiatry during the past twenty-five years has presented much data suggesting that the form models take is in fact far more strongly determined by a child's actual experiences throughout childhood than was formerly supposed. This is a field of vital interest and calls urgently for skilled investigation. A particular clinical and research problem is that disturbed individuals seem often to maintain within themselves more than one working model both of the world and of the self in it. Such multiple models, moreover, are frequently incompatible with each other and can be more or less unconscious.

Enough perhaps has been said to show that the concept of working models is central to the schema proposed. The concept can be elaborated to enable many aspects of personality structure and internal world to be described in ways that permit precision and rigorous research.

Thus the theory advanced here is not only couched in different language but contains a number of concepts distinct from those of traditional theory. Amongst many other things, these concepts enable a fresh approach to be made to the age-long problem of separation anxiety which, when excessive, is inimical to the development of self-reliance.

THE PROBLEM OF SEPARATION ANXIETY

The many observations of the behaviour of young children when removed from their parents and placed in strange surroundings with strange people, described by James Robertson and others during the past twenty years, have still not been fully articulated into clinical theory. There is still no agreement on why the experience should be so distressing to a child at the time, nor why afterwards he should be so intensely apprehensive lest it happen again.

During recent years a number of experiments have been conducted on young monkeys in which they are separated from mother, usually for about one week. Whatever differences there may prove to be between the responses of monkeys and humans in such a situation, what is immediately striking is the similarity of response. In most species of monkey studied, protest at separation and depression during it are very pronounced, and, after reunion, clinging to mother is much increased. During the subsequent months, though individuals vary, the separated infants tend on average to explore less and to cling more; and they remain detectably more timid than young monkeys that have not had a separation. (For a review of these findings see Hinde and Spencer-Booth 1971.)

These monkey studies are of great value in that:

(a) They provide clear evidence from planned experiments that hold stable many variables that in real life observations of humans make firm conclusions difficult to draw;

(b) They demonstrate that, even when all other variables are held constant, a period of separation from mother elicits protest and depression during the separation and much increased separation anxiety after it;

(c) They make it clear that the kinds of response to separation that are seen in humans can in other species be mediated at a primitive, and presumably infra-symbolic, level.

This last finding calls in question the various clinically derived theories that seek to explain separation anxiety, since most of them take it virtually for granted that involuntary separation from a mother-figure cannot of itself elicit anxiety or fear and that there must therefore be some other danger that is foreseen and feared. Many and diverse suggestions have been advanced of what this other danger might be. For example, Freud (1926), who from the first regarded separation anxiety as a key problem, suggested that for humans the ultimate 'danger-situation is a recognized, remembered, expected situation of helplessness'. Melanie Klein has advanced theories invoking a death instinct and fear of annihilation, and also theories deriving from her views about depressive and persecutory anxiety. Birth trauma is yet another suggestion. On reading the literature it is abundantly clear that many of the most strenuously debated issues in psychopathology and psychotherapy have turned, and still turn, on how we conceptualize the origin and nature of separation anxiety (Bowlby 1960a, 1961a, 1973). Since the debate has been going on for so long and with so little progress the question is raised whether the wrong questions are being asked and/or the wrong initial assumptions made. Let us examine, therefore, what the initial assumptions have been.

Almost all theory about what arouses fear and anxiety in humans has started from the assumption that fear is aroused appropriately only in situations that are perceived as intrinsically painful or dangerous. Such perception is thought to derive either from previous experience of pain or else from some innate awareness of dangerous forces within. One or other of these assumptions is to be found in learning theory, in traditional psychiatry, as exemplified for example in a paper by Lewis (1967), and in all the various versions of psychoanalysis and its derivatives.

Anyone who adopts an assumption of this sort is, of course, very quickly faced with the fact that human beings frequently show fear in a number of common situations that do not seem inherently painful or dangerous. How many of us, it may be asked, would relish entering a completely strange house in the dark on our own? What a relief it would be were we to have a companion with us, or had a good light, or preferably both companion and light. Although it is during childhood that situations of this sort elicit fear most readily and intensely, it is idle to pretend that adults are above such things. To refer to fears of these kinds as 'infantile', as is often done, begs a lot of questions.

It is striking how few empirical studies there have been of the situations that commonly arouse fear in humans since Jersild's systematic work of the early thirties. The publications in which they are reported (e.g., Jersild and Holmes 1935; Jersild 1943) are mines of useful information.

In children between the second and fifth years of life, Jersild reports, there are a number of well-defined situations that commonly elicit fear. For example, records of 136 children over a three-week period show that not less than 40 per cent of them showed fear, on one occasion at least, when confronted with *each* of the following: (a) noise and events associated with noise, (b) height, (c) strange people, or familiar people in strange guise, (d) strange objects and situations, (e) animals, (f) pain or persons associated with pain.

There was also abundant evidence that children showed less fear when accompanied by an adult than when alone. To anyone familiar with children these findings are hardly revolutionary.

Yet it is not easy to square them with the assumptions from which most theorizing starts. Freud was keenly alive to the problem and confessed himself perplexed. Amongst the solutions he tried was his well-known attempt to distinguish between a real danger and an unknown danger. The argument he advances in *Inhibitions, Symptoms and Anxiety* (1926) can be put in a nutshell, using his own words. 'A real danger is a danger which threatens a person from an external object.' Whenever anxiety is 'about a known danger', therefore, it can be regarded as 'realistic anxiety'; whereas whenever it is 'about an unknown danger' it is to be regarded as 'neurotic anxiety'. Since fears of being alone, in the dark or with strangers are, in Freud's view, about unknown dangers they are to be judged neurotic (*Standard Edition* Vol. 20, pp. 165–7). Because all children experience such fears, moreover, all children are held to suffer from neurosis (pp. 147–8). There must be many who find themselves dissatisfied with this solution.

The difficulties Freud struggled with disappear when a comparative approach to human fear is adopted. For it becomes evident that man is by no means the only species to show fear in situations that are not intrinsically painful or dangerous (Hinde 1970). Animals of very many species show fear behaviour in response to noise and other sudden changes of stimulation, to darkness, and also to strangers and strange events. The visual cliff and a stimulus that rapidly expands also regularly elicit fear in animals of a number of species.

When we ask how it has come about that situations of these sorts should so readily elicit fear in animals of so many species, it is not difficult to see that, whilst none of them is intrinsically dangerous, each is in some degree potentially dangerous. Put in another way, whilst none may carry a high risk of danger, each carries a slightly increased risk of danger, even if the risk is increased, say, only from 1 per cent to 5 per cent.

Looked at in this light each of these fear-arousing situations is seen to be a natural clue to an increased risk of danger. To respond with fear to all such situations is therefore to reduce risks. Because such behaviour has survival value, the argument runs, the genetic equipment of a species becomes such that each member of it at birth is biased to develop so that it usually comes to behave in these typical ways. Man is no exception.

A distinction that is invoked here that is a commonplace for ethologists but a source of much confusion and perplexity amongst psychologists, both experimental and clinical, is the distinction between causation and biological function – the distinction between, on the one hand, what conditions elicit behaviour and, on the other, what contribution to species survival such behaviour may make. In this theory strangeness and the other natural clues is each regarded as playing a causal role in eliciting fear behaviour; whilst the function of such behaviour is protection.

Perhaps the distinction between the cause and the function of a piece of behaviour can be clarified by reference to sexual behaviour in which the distinction is so patently obvious that it is usually taken for granted and virtually forgotten. Spelled out the distinction runs as follows: hormonal states of the organism and certain characteristics of the partner, together, lead to sexual interest and play causal roles in eliciting sexual behaviour. The biological function of that behaviour however is another matter; it is reproduction. Because causation and function are distinct, it is possible, by means of contraception, to intervene between the behaviour and the function it serves.

In animals of all non-human species behaviour is engaged in without the animal (presumably) having any insight whatever into function. The same is true also of most humans most of the time. Seen in this light there is nothing to surprise us that humans should habitually respond with fear behaviour in certain situations despite the fact that an external observer might know that in such situations risk to life is only marginally increased, or even not increased at all. What a person responds to initially is simply the situation – sudden change of noise or light level, a strange face or strange happening, sudden movement – not to any estimate of risk. Sober calculation of risk may or may not follow.

Unwilling separation of young from parent, or for that matter of adult from trusted companion, can be regarded simply as another situation of the same sort, although rather a special example of it. Even in civilized communities there are many circumstances in which the risk of danger is somewhat greater when one is alone than when with a companion. This is especially so during childhood. For example, risk of accidents in the home are obviously greater when a child is left alone than when his mother or father is around. The same is true of accidents in the streets. During 1968 in the London Borough of Southwark, 46 per cent of all traffic accidents happened to children under fifteen, with the highest incidence in the age-group three to nine. More than 60 per cent of these children were entirely alone and two-thirds of the remainder in the company only of another child. For the elderly or sick, living alone is a notorious hazard. Even for healthy adult males to go hill-walking or climbing alone is materially to increase risk to life. In the environment in which man evolved, the risks attendant on being alone are likely to have been much greater. Reflection shows therefore that, because being alone increases risk, there is good reason why man should have evolved behavioural systems that lead him to avoid it. For humans to respond with fear to loss of a trusted companion is thus no more puzzling than that he should respond with fear to any of the other natural clues to potential danger – strangeness, sudden movement, sudden change in noise or light level. In every case to respond so has survival value.

A very special feature of fear behaviour both in humans and other animals is the degree to which it is increased in situations characterized by the presence of two or more of the natural clues; for example, the stranger who suddenly approaches, the strange dog that barks, the unexpected noise heard in the dark. Commenting on the twenty-one-day observations made by parents of fear-arousing situations, Jersild and Holmes (1935) note that combinations of two or more of the following features were frequently reported to be present *together*: noise, strange people and situations, the dark, sudden and unexpected movement, and being alone. Whereas a situation characterized by a single one of these features might only alert, fear, more or less intense, may well be aroused when several are present together.

Because the response to a combination of factors is often so dramatically greater than, or different to, what it is to any one singly, it is convenient to refer to such situations as 'compound', a term chosen to echo the chemical analogue (Bowlby 1973).

In keeping with other findings on the effects of compound situations, experiments both with human children and with rhesus monkeys (Rowell and Hinde 1963) show what a tremendous difference to the intensity of fear responses is made by the presence or absence of a trusted companion. For example, Jersild and Holmes (1935) found that, when children in their third and fourth years were asked to go alone to find a ball that had gone down a dark passage, half refused to do so despite encouragement from the experimenter. When the experimenter accompanied them, however, almost all were ready to do it. Differences of a similar kind were seen in a number of other slightly frightening situations, for example, when a child was asked to approach and pat a large dog brought in on a lead.

These findings are so much in keeping with common experience that it may seem absurd to labour them. Yet, it is evident that, when psychologists and psychiatrists come to theorize about fear and anxiety, the significance of these phenomena is gravely underestimated. For example, when due attention is paid to these findings it ceases to be a mystery that, in all but very familiar situations, fear and anxiety are greatly reduced by the mere presence of a trusted companion. These findings enable us to understand also why the accessibility of parents and their willingness to respond provides an infant, a child, an adolescent, and a young adult with conditions in which he feels secure and with a base from which he feels confident to explore. They cast light too on the way that, from adolescence onwards, other trusted figures can come to provide similar services.

This brings the argument full circle and helps to explain how it comes about that strong and consistent support from parents, combined with encouragement and respect for a child's autonomy, so far from sapping self-reliance, provide the conditions in which it can best grow. It helps to explain, too, why, conversely, an experience of separation or loss, or threats of separation or loss, especially when used by parents as sanctions for good behaviour, can undermine a child's trust both in others and in himself, and so lead to one or another deviation from optimum development – to lack of self-confidence, to chronic anxiety or depression, to aloof non-committal, or to defiant independence that has a hollow ring.

A well-based self-reliance, we may conclude, is usually the product of slow and unchecked growth from infancy into maturity during which, through interaction with trustworthy and encouraging others, a person learns how to combine trust in others with trust in himself.

NOTES

1   More recent publications by Dr. Salter Ainsworth and her colleagues are to be found in a review paper by Ainsworth (1977) and in a definitive monograph, Ainsworth *et al.* (1978).

2   See the objections to this phraseology in note 1 to Chapter 3. A better way of phrasing this passage would be: '. . ., that attachment behaviour is elicited most readily during the second and third years of life and persists indefinitely, though in healthy development it is elicited less readily, . . .'

7

THE MAKING AND BREAKING OF AFFECTIONAL BONDS*

Each year the Royal College of Psychiatrists arranges a lecture to be given in honour of Henry Maudsley, who was a benefactor of the College's predecessor, the Royal Medico-Psychological Association (and also of the Maudsley Hospital). I was invited to give the 1976 lecture at the meeting of the College held in London during the autumn. It was published in much amplified form and in two parts the following spring.

AETIOLOGY AND PSYCHOPATHOLOGY IN THE LIGHT OF ATTACHMENT THEORY

From the time when I first studied psychiatry at the Maudsley Hospital my interests have centred on the contribution that a person's environment makes to his psychological development. For many years this was a neglected area and it is only now that

---

* Originally published in British Journal of Psychiatry (1977) **130**: 201–10 and 421–31. Reprinted by permission of the Royal College of Psychiatrists.

it is receiving the attention it deserves. That is no fault of that staunch advocate of the scientific study of mental disorder whose life and work we remember today. For, although from some passages in his writings it might be thought that Henry Maudsley gave little weight to environmental factors, this is far from being true as a reading of his influential book, *Responsibility in Mental Diseases*, first published almost exactly a century ago, makes clear. Indeed, from the very start of his career Maudsley's approach was that of the biologist – as we might expect in a farmer's son; and he knew that in psychiatry as in all things biological it is necessary to consider both 'the subject and his environment, the man and his circumstances' and that that requires we adopt a developmental approach.* Thus, in preparing this lecture, which I feel much honoured to have been invited to give, I have felt sustained by the belief that its theme, that of social and emotional development within different types of family environment, is in keeping with all that Henry Maudsley stood for.

What for convenience I am terming attachment theory is a way of conceptualizing the propensity of human beings to make strong affectional bonds to particular others and of explaining the many forms of emotional distress and personality disturbance, including anxiety, anger, depression, and emotional detachment, to which unwilling separation and loss give rise. As a body of theory it deals with the same phenomena that hitherto have been dealt with in terms of 'dependency need' or of 'object relations' or of 'symbiosis and individuation'. Though it incorporates much psychoanalytic thinking, the theory differs from traditional psychoanalysis in adopting a number of principles that

* The quotation is from an essay by Maudsley published in 1860. For this and other information regarding Maudsley's life and work I am indebted to the account given by Sir Aubrey Lewis in his twenty-fifth Maudsley Lecture (Lewis 1951).

derive from the relatively new disciplines of ethology and control theory; by so doing it is enabled to dispense with concepts of psychic energy and drive and also to forge close links with cognitive psychology. Merits claimed for it are that whilst its concepts are psychological they are compatible with those of neurophysiology and developmental biology and also that it conforms to the ordinary criteria of a scientific discipline.

Advocates of attachment theory argue that many forms of psychiatric disturbance can be attributed either to deviations in the development of attachment behaviour or, more rarely, to failure of its development; and also that the theory casts light on both the origin and the treatment of these conditions. Put briefly, the thesis of this lecture is that if we are to help such a patient therapeutically it is necessary that we enable him to consider in detail how his present modes of perceiving and dealing with emotionally significant persons, including the therapist, may be being influenced and perhaps seriously distorted by the experiences which he had with his parents during the years of his childhood and adolescence, and some of which may perhaps be continuing into the present. This entails his reviewing those experiences in as honest a way as possible, a review which the therapist can either assist or impede. In a brief account it is possible only to state principles and the rationale behind them. We start with a brief sketch of what is meant by attachment theory. (For a fuller description of the data on which it is based, the concepts employed and the arguments in its favour, with full references, see the two volumes of *Attachment and Loss* now published, Bowlby 1969, 1973.)

Until the mid nineteen-fifties only one explicitly formulated view of the nature and origin of affectional bonds was prevalent, and in this matter there was agreement between psychoanalysts and learning theorists. Bonds between individuals develop, it was held, because an individual discovers that, in order to reduce certain drives, e.g., for food in infancy and for sex in adult life, another human being is necessary. This type of theory postulates two kinds of drive, primary and secondary; it categorizes food and sex as primary and 'dependency' and other personal relationships as secondary. Although object relations theorists (Balint, Fairbairn, Guntrip, Klein, Winnicott) have tried to modify this formulation, the concepts of dependency, orality, and regression have persisted.

Studies of the ill-effects on personality development of deprivation of maternal care led me to question the adequacy of the traditional model. Early in the nineteen-fifties Lorenz's work on imprinting, which had first appeared in 1935, became more generally known and offered an alternative approach. At least in some species of bird, he had found, strong bonds to a mother-figure develop during the early days of life without any reference to food and simply through the young being exposed to and becoming familiar with the figure in question. Arguing that the empirical data on the development of a human child's tie to his mother can be understood better in terms of a model derived from ethology I outlined a theory of attachment in a paper published in 1958. Simultaneously and independently, Harlow (1958) published the results of his first studies of infant rhesus monkeys reared on dummy-mothers. A young monkey, he found, will cling to a dummy that does not feed it provided the dummy is soft and comfortable to cling to.

During the past fifteen years the results of a number of empirical studies of human children have been published (e.g., Robertson and Robertson 1967–72; Heinicke and Westheimer 1966; Ainsworth 1967; Ainsworth, Bell, and Stayton 1971, 1974; Blurton Jones 1972), theory has been greatly amplified (e.g., Ainsworth 1969; Bowlby 1969; Bischof 1975), and the relationship of attachment theory to dependency theory examined (Maccoby and Masters 1970; Gewirtz 1972).[1] New formulations regarding pathological anxiety and phobia have been advanced (Bowlby 1973) and also regarding mourning and its psychiatric complications (e.g., Bowlby 1961c; Parkes 1965, 1971a, 1972). Parkes (1971b) has extended the theory to cover the range of responses seen whenever a person encounters a major change in his life situation. Many studies have been made of comparable behaviour in primate species (see review by Hinde 1974).

Briefly put, attachment behaviour is conceived as any form of behaviour that results in a person attaining or retaining proximity to some other differentiated and preferred individual, who is usually conceived as stronger and/or wiser. Whilst especially evident during early childhood, attachment behaviour is held to characterize human beings from the cradle to the grave. It includes crying and calling, which elicit care, following and clinging, and also strong protest should a child be left alone or with strangers. With age the frequency and the intensity with which such behaviour is exhibited diminish steadily. Nevertheless, all these forms of behaviour persist as an important part of man's behavioural equipment. In adults they are especially evident when a person is distressed, ill, or afraid. The particular patterns of attachment behaviour shown by an individual turn partly on his present age, sex, and circumstances and partly on the experiences he has had with attachment figures earlier in his life.

As a way of conceptualizing proximity keeping, attachment theory, in contrast to dependency theory, emphasizes the following features:*

(a) *Specificity* Attachment behaviour is directed towards one or a few specific individuals, usually in clear order of preference.

(b) *Duration* An attachment endures, usually for a large part of the life cycle. Although during adolescence early attachments

* In describing these features I am drawing on the text of an article (Bowlby 1975) written for Volume 6 of the *American Handbook of Psychiatry* © 1975 by Basic Books Inc., and am grateful to the editors and publishers for permission to do so.

may attenuate and become supplemented by new ones, and in some cases are replaced by them, early attachments are not easily abandoned and they commonly persist.

(c) *Engagement of emotion** Many of the most intense emotions arise during the formation, the maintenance, the disruption, and the renewal of attachment relationships. The formation of a bond is described as falling in love, maintaining a bond as loving someone, and losing a partner as grieving over someone. Similarly, threat of loss arouses anxiety and actual loss gives rise to sorrow; whilst each of these situations is likely to arouse anger. The unchallenged maintenance of a bond is experienced as a source of security and the renewal of a bond as a source of joy. Because such emotions are usually a reflection of the state of a person's affectional bonds, the psychology and psychopathology of emotion is found to be in large part the psychology and psychopathology of affectional bonds.

(d) *Ontogeny* In the great majority of human infants attachment behaviour to a preferred figure develops during the first nine months of life. The more experience of social interaction an infant has with a person the more likely is he to become attached to that person. For this reason, whoever is principally mothering a child becomes his principal attachment figure. Attachment behaviour remains readily activated until near the end of the third year; in healthy development it becomes gradually less readily activated thereafter.

(e) *Learning* Whereas learning to distinguish the familiar from the strange is a key process in the development of attachment, the conventional rewards and punishments used by experimental psychologists play only a small part. Indeed, an attachment can develop despite repeated punishment from the attachment figure.

* Although this paragraph is little different to similar paragraphs in Chapter 4 and 6 I am leaving it unchanged because without it this Lecture would be seriously incomplete.

(f) *Organization* Initially attachment behaviour is mediated by responses organized on fairly simple lines. From the end of the first year, it becomes mediated by increasingly sophisticated behavioural systems organized cybernetically and incorporating representational models of the environment and self. These systems are activated by certain conditions and terminated by others. Amongst activating conditions are strangeness, hunger, fatigue, and anything frightening. Terminating conditions include sight or sound of mother-figure and, especially, happy interaction with her. When attachment behaviour is strongly aroused, termination may require touching or clinging to her and/or being cuddled by her. Conversely, when mother-figure is present or her whereabouts well-known, a child ceases to show attachment behaviour and, instead, explores his environment.

(g) *Biological function* Attachment behaviour occurs in the young of almost all species of mammal, and in a number of species it persists throughout adult life. Although there are many differences of detail between species, maintenance of proximity by an immature animal to a preferred adult, almost always mother, is the rule, which suggests that such behaviour has survival value. Elsewhere (Bowlby 1969) I have argued that by far the most likely function of attachment behaviour is protection, mainly from predators.

Thus attachment behaviour is conceived as a class of behaviour distinct from feeding behaviour and sexual behaviour and of at least an equal significance in human life. There is nothing intrinsically childish or pathological about it.

It will be noted that the concept of attachment differs greatly from that of dependence. For example, dependence is not specifically related to maintenance of proximity, it is not directed towards a specific individual, it does not imply an enduring bond, nor is it necessarily associated with strong feeling. No biological function is attributed to it. Furthermore, in the concept of dependence there are value implications the exact opposite of those that the concept of attachment conveys. Whereas to refer to a person as dependent tends to be disparaging, to describe him as attached to someone can well be an expression of approval. Conversely, for a person to be detached in his personal relations is usually regarded as less than admirable. The disparaging element in the concept of dependence, which reflects a failure to recognize the value that attachment behaviour has for survival, is held to be a fatal weakness to its clinical use.

In what follows, the individual who shows attachment behaviour is usually referred to as child and the attachment figure as mother. This is because the behaviour has so far only been closely studied in children. What is said, however, is held to apply also to adults and to whoever is acting for them as their attachment figure – often a spouse, sometimes a parent, and more often than might be supposed a child.

It was remarked (under (f) above) that when mother is present or her whereabouts well-known and is willing to take part in friendly interchange, a child usually ceases to show attachment behaviour and, instead, explores his environment. In such a situation mother can be regarded as providing her child with a secure base from which to explore and to which he can return, especially should he become tired or frightened. Throughout the rest of a person's life he is likely to show the same pattern of behaviour, moving away from those he loves for ever-increasing distances and lengths of time yet always maintaining contact and sooner or later returning. The base from which an adult operates is likely to be either his family of origin or else a new base which he has created for himself. Anyone who has no such base is rootless and intensely lonely.

In the account given so far two patterns of behaviour other than attachment have been referred to, namely exploration and care-giving.

There is now a mass of evidence to support the view that exploratory activity is of great importance in its own right, enabling a person or an animal to build up a coherent picture of environmental features which may at any time become of importance for survival. Children and other young creatures are notoriously curious and inquiring, which commonly leads them to move away from their attachment figure. In this sense exploratory behaviour is antithetical to attachment behaviour. In healthy individuals the two kinds of behaviour normally alternate.

The behaviour of parents, and of anyone else in a care-giving role, is complementary to attachment behaviour. The roles of the care-giver are first to be available and responsive as and when wanted and, second, to intervene judiciously should the child or older person who is being cared for be heading for trouble. Not only is it a key role but there is substantial evidence that how it is discharged by a person's parents determines in great degree whether or not he grows up to be mentally healthy. For that reason and also because it is the role we fill when we act as psychotherapists, our understanding of it is held to be of central importance to the practice of psychotherapy.

One further point needs to be made before we consider the implications of this schema for a theory of aetiology and psychopathology and thence for the practice of psychotherapy. It concerns our understanding of anxiety and of separation anxiety in particular.

A common assumption that runs through most psychiatric and psycho-pathological theory is that fear should be manifested only in situations that are truly dangerous, and that fear shown in any other situation is neurotic. This leads to the conclusion that, because separation from an attachment figure cannot be regarded as a truly dangerous situation, anxiety over separation from that figure is neurotic. Examination of the evidence shows that both the assumption and the conclusion to which it leads are false.

When approached empirically separation from an attachment figure is found to be one of a class of situations each of which is likely to elicit fear but none of which can be regarded as intrinsically dangerous. These situations comprise, amongst others, darkness, sudden large changes of stimulus level including loud noises, sudden movement, strange people, and strange things. Evidence shows that animals of many species are alarmed by such situations (Hinde 1970), and that this is true of human children (Jersild 1947) and also of adults. Furthermore, fear is especially likely to be elicited when two or more of these conditions are present simultaneously, for example, hearing a loud noise when alone in the dark.

The explanation of why individuals should so regularly respond to these situations with fear is held to be that, whilst none of the situations is intrinsically dangerous, each carries with it an *increased risk* of danger. Noise, strangeness, isolation, and, for many species, darkness, all these are conditions statistically associated with an increased risk of danger. Noise may presage a natural disaster – fire, flood, or landslide. To a young animal a predator is strange, it moves, and it often strikes at night, and it is far more likely to do so when the potential victim is alone. Because to behave so promotes both survival and breeding success, the theory runs, the young of species that have survived, including man, are found to be genetically biased so to develop that they respond to the properties of noise, strangeness, sudden approach, and darkness by taking avoiding action or running away – they behave in fact as though danger were actually present. In a comparable way they respond to isolation by seeking company. Fear responses elicited by such naturally occurring clues to danger are a part of man's basic behavioural equipment (Bowlby 1973).

Seen in this light anxiety over unwilling separation from an attachment figure resembles the anxiety that the general of an expeditionary force feels when communications with his base are cut or threatened.

This leads to the conclusion that anxiety over an unwilling separation can be a perfectly normal and healthy reaction. What may be puzzling is why such anxiety is aroused in some people at such very high intensity or, conversely, in others, at such low intensities. This brings us to questions of aetiology and psychopathology.

Throughout this century debate has raged about the role of childhood experiences in the causation of psychiatric disturbance. Not only have traditionally minded psychiatrists been sceptical of their relevance but psychoanalysts have been at sixes and sevens about them. For long, most analysts who have thought real-life experience to be of importance concentrated attention on the first two or three years of life and on certain techniques of baby care – the ways an infant is fed or toilet trained – and whether he witnesses parental intercourse. Attention to family interaction and the particular way a parent treats a particular child was not encouraged. Some extremists, indeed, have held that the systematic study of a person's experiences within his family lie outside the proper interest of a psychoanalyst.

No one engaged in child psychiatry, better termed family psychiatry, can possibly share such a view. In a great majority of cases not only is there evidence of disturbed family relationships but the emotional problems of the parents, derived from their own unhappy childhoods, commonly loom large. Thus the problem has always seemed to me not whether to study a patient's family environment but to decide what features are likely to be relevant, what methods of inquiry are practicable, and what type of theory best fits the data. Because many others have adopted the same view a great deal of reasonably reliable research has now been done by workers of many disciplines. It is from the results of this research, interpreted in terms of attachment theory, that I offer the generalizations and views that follow.

The key point of my thesis is that there is a strong causal

relationship between an individual's experiences with his parents and his later capacity to make affectional bonds, and that certain common variations in that capacity, manifesting themselves in marital problems and trouble with children as well as in neurotic symptoms and personality disorders, can be attributed to certain common variations in the ways that parents perform their roles. Much of the evidence on which the thesis rests is reviewed in the second volume of *Attachment and Loss* (Chapter 15 onwards). The main variable to which I draw attention is the extent to which a child's parents (a) provide him with a secure base and (b) encourage him to explore from it. In these roles the performance of parents varies along several parameters of which perhaps the most important, because it pervades all relations, is the extent to which parents recognize and respect a child's desire for a secure base and his need of it, and shape their behaviour accordingly. This entails, first, an intuitive and sympathetic understanding of a child's attachment behaviour and a willingness to meet it and thereby terminate it, and, second, recognition that one of the commonest sources of a child's anger is the frustration of his desire for love and care, and that his anxiety commonly reflects uncertainty whether parents will continue to be available. Complementary in importance to a parent's respect for a child's attachment desires is respect for his desire to explore and gradually to extend his relationships both with peers and with other adults.

Research suggests that in many areas of Britain and the United States rather more than half the child population is growing up with parents who are providing their children with such conditions. Typically these children grow up to be secure and self-reliant, and to be trusting, cooperative, and helpful towards others. In the psychoanalytic literature such a person is said to have a strong ego; and he may be described as showing 'basic trust' (Erikson 1950), 'mature dependence' (Fairbairn 1952) or as having 'introjected a good object' (Klein 1948). In terms of attachment theory he is described as having built up a representational model of himself as being both able to help himself and as worthy of being helped should difficulties arise.

By contrast, many children (in some populations one-third or more) grow up with parents who do not provide these conditions. Note here that the focus of attention is on the particular relationship a parent has with a particular child, since parents do not treat every child alike and may provide excellent conditions for one and very adverse ones for another.

Let us consider some of the more common deviant patterns of attachment behaviour that are shown by adolescents and also by adults, with examples of typical childhood experiences which those who show them are likely to have had and may still be having.

Many of those referred to psychiatrists are anxious, insecure individuals, usually described as over-dependent or immature. Under stress they are apt to develop neurotic symptoms, depression, or phobia. Research shows them to have been exposed to at least one, and usually more than one, of certain typical patterns of pathogenic parenting, which include:

(a) one or both parents being persistently unresponsive to the child's care-eliciting behaviour and/or actively disparaging and rejecting him;

(b) discontinuities of parenting, occurring more or less frequently, including periods in hospital or institution;

(c) persistent threats by parents not to love a child, used as a means of controlling him;

(d) threats by parents to abandon the family, used either as a method of disciplining the child or as a way of coercing a spouse;

(e) threats by one parent either to desert or even to kill the other or else to commit suicide (each of them more common than might be supposed);

(f) inducing a child to feel guilty by claiming that his behaviour is or will be responsible for the parent's illness or death.

Any of these experiences can lead a child, an adolescent or an adult to live in constant anxiety lest he lose his attachment figure and, as a result, to have a low threshold for manifesting attachment behaviour. The condition is best described as one of anxious attachment.*

An additional set of conditions to which some such individuals have been, and may still be, exposed is that of a parent, usually mother, exerting pressure on them to act as an attachment figure for her, thus inverting the normal relationship. Means of exerting such pressure vary from the unconscious encouragement of a premature sense of responsibility for others to the deliberate use of threats or induction of guilt. Individuals treated in these ways are likely to become over-conscientious and guilt-ridden as well as anxiously attached. A majority of cases of school phobia and agoraphobia arise probably in this way.

All the variants of parental behaviour so far described are likely not only to arouse a child's anger against his parents but to inhibit its expression. The result is much partially unconscious resentment, which persists into adult life and is expressed usually in a direction away from the parents and towards someone weaker, e.g., a spouse or a child. Such a person is likely to be subject also to strong unconscious yearnings for love and support which may express themselves in some aberrant form of care-eliciting behaviour, for example, half-hearted suicide attempts, conversion symptoms, anorexia nervosa, hypochondria (Henderson 1974).

A pattern of attachment behaviour that is overtly the opposite of anxious attachment is one described by Parkes (1973) as that of compulsive self-reliance. So far from seeking the love and care

* There is no evidence whatever for the traditional idea, still widespread, that such a person has been overindulged as a child and so has grown up 'spoilt'.

of others a person who exhibits this pattern insists on keeping a stiff upper lip and doing everything for himself whatever the conditions. These people too are apt to crack under stress and to present with psychosomatic symptoms or depression.

Many such persons have had experiences not unlike those of individuals who develop anxious attachment; but they have reacted to them differently by inhibiting attachment feeling and behaviour and disclaiming, perhaps even mocking, any desire for close relations with anyone who might provide love and care. It requires no great insight to realize, however, that they are deeply distrustful of close relationships and terrified of allowing themselves to rely on anyone else, in some cases in order to avoid the pain of being rejected and in others to avoid being subjected to pressure to become someone else's caretaker. As in the case of anxious attachment, there is likely to be much underlying resentment which, when elicited, is directed against weaker persons, and also unexpressed yearning for love and support.

A pattern of attachment behaviour related to compulsive self-reliance is that of compulsive care-giving. A person showing it may engage in many close relationships but always in the role of giving care, never that of receiving it. Often the one selected is a lame duck who may for a time welcome the care bestowed. But the compulsive care-giver will also strive to care for those who neither seek nor welcome it. The typical childhood experience of such people is to have a mother who, due to depression or some other disability, was unable to care for the child but, instead, welcomed being cared for and perhaps also demanded help in caring for younger siblings. Thus, from early childhood, the person who develops in this way has found that the only affectional bond available is one in which he must always be the care-giver and that the only care he can ever receive is the care he gives himself. (Children growing up in institutions some-times develop in this way, too.) Here again, as in the case of the compulsively self-reliant, there is much latent yearning for love and care and much latent anger with the parents for not having provided it; and, once again, much anxiety and guilt about expressing such desires. Winnicott (1965) has described individuals of this sort as having developed a 'false self' and agrees that its origin is to be found in the person not having received 'good enough' mothering as a child. To assist such a person to discover his 'true self' entails helping him recognize and become possessed of his yearning for love and care and his anger at those who earlier failed to give it him.

Life events that are especially liable to act as stressors for individuals whose attachment and care-giving behaviour has developed along one or other of the lines so far described are the serious illness or death either of an attachment figure or of someone cared for, or some other form of separation from them. A serious illness intensifies anxiety and perhaps guilt. Death or separation confirm the person's worst expectations and lead to despair as well as anxiety. In these people mourning a death or a separation is likely to take an atypical course. In the case of the anxiously attached, mourning is likely to be characterized by unusually intense anger and/or self-reproach, with depression, and to persist for much longer than normal. In the case of the compulsively self-reliant, mourning may be delayed for months or years. None the less strain and irritability are usually present and episodic depressions may occur, but often so long a time later that the causal connection with the death or separation is lost to sight. These pathological forms of mourning are discussed by Parkes (1972).

Not only are people of the kind so far described likely to break down after a loss or separation, but they are likely to encounter certain typical difficulties when they get married and have children. In relation to a marriage partner, a person may exhibit anxious attachment and make constant demands for love and care; or else he or she may exhibit compulsive care-giving to the other with latent resentment that it seems neither appreciated nor reciprocated. In relation to a child, also, either of these patterns may be exhibited. In the first case the parent requires the child to be his or her caregiver and in the second insists on providing him with care even when it is no longer appropriate, which results in 'smother love'.* Disturbances of parenting behaviour result also from a parent perceiving and treating his child as though the child were one of his siblings which can result, for example, in a father being jealous of the attentions his wife gives their child.

Another common form of disturbance is when a parent perceives his child as a replica of himself, especially of those aspects of himself which he has endeavoured to stamp out, and strives then to stamp them out in his child also. In these efforts he is likely to use a version of the same methods of discipline – perhaps crude and violent, perhaps censorious or sarcastic, perhaps guilt-inducing – to which he himself was subjected as a child and which resulted in his developing the very problems he is now striving so inappropriately to prevent or cure in his child. A husband can also perceive and treat his wife in the same way. Similarly, a wife and mother can adopt this pattern in her perception and treatment of her husband or child. When confronted by disagreeable and self-defeating behaviour of this sort it is useful to remember that each of us is apt to do unto others as we have been done by. The bullying adult is the bullied child grown bigger.

When one adopts either towards oneself or towards others the

---

* The term 'symbiotic' is sometimes used to describe these suffocatingly close relationships. The term is not happily chosen, however, since in biology it refers to a mutually advantageous partnership between two organisms whereas the family relationships so termed are seriously maladaptive. To describe the child as 'over-protected' is equally misleading since it fails to recognize the insistent demands for care that the parent is putting on the child.

same attitudes and forms of behaviour that one's own parent adopted and may still be adopting towards oneself one can be said to be identifying with that parent. The processes by which such attitudes and forms of behaviour are acquired are presumably those of observational learning and thus no different to those by which other complex forms of behaviour, including useful skills, are acquired.

Of the many other patterns of disturbed family functioning and personality development that can be understood in terms of the pathological development of attachment behaviour, a well-known one is the emotionally detached individual who is incapable of maintaining a stable affectional bond with anyone. People with this disability may be labelled as psychopathic and/or hysterical. They are often delinquent and suicidal. The typical history is one of prolonged deprivation of maternal care during the earliest years of life, usually combined with later rejection and/or threats of rejection by parents or foster parents.*

To explain why individuals of different sorts should continue to exhibit the characteristics described long after they have grown up, it seems necessary to postulate that whatever representational models of attachment figures and of self an individual builds during his childhood and adolescence, tend to persist relatively unchanged into and throughout adult life. As a result he tends to assimilate any new person with whom he may form a bond, such as spouse or child, or employer or therapist, to an existing model (either of one or other parent or of self), and often to continue to do so despite repeated evidence that the model is

---

* Since all the psychiatric conditions referred to represent varying degrees and patterns of the same underlying psychopathology there is no more prospect of distinguishing one sharply from another than there is of distinguishing sharply between different forms of tuberculous infection. In accounting for the differences, genetic factors as well as variations in the experiences of different individuals are likely to be relevant.

inappropriate. Similarly, he expects to be perceived and treated by them in ways that would be appropriate to his self-model, and to continue with such expectations despite contrary evidence. Such biased perceptions and expectations lead to various misconceived beliefs about the other people, to false expectations about the way they will behave and to inappropriate actions, intended to forestall their expected behaviour. Thus, to take a simple example, a man who during childhood was frequently threatened with abandonment can easily attribute such intentions to his wife. He will then misinterpret things she says or does in terms of such intent, and then take whatever action he thinks would best meet the situation he believes to exist. Misunderstanding and conflict must follow. In all this he is as unaware that he is being biased by his past experience as he is that his present beliefs and expectations are mistaken.

In traditional theory the processes described are often referred to in terms of 'internalizing a problem' and the misattributions and misperceptions ascribed to projection, introjection, or fantasy. Not only are the resulting statements apt to be ambiguous but the fact that such misattributions and misperceptions are directly derived from previous real-life experience is either only vaguely alluded to or else totally obscured. By framing the processes in terms of cognitive psychology, I believe, much greater precision becomes possible and hypotheses regarding the causative role of different sorts of childhood experience, through the persistence of representational models of attachment figures and self at an unconscious level, can be formulated in testable form.

It should be noted that inappropriate but persistent representational models often co-exist with more appropriate ones. For example, a husband may oscillate between believing his wife to be loyal to him and suspecting her of plans to desert. Clinical experience suggests that the stronger the emotions aroused in a relationship the more likely are the earlier and less conscious models to become dominant. To account for such mental functioning, which is traditionally discussed in terms of defensive processes, presents a challenge to cognitive psychologists but one to which they are already addressing themselves (e.g., Erdelyi 1974).[2]

SOME PRINCIPLES OF PSYCHOTHERAPY

Such then are the elements of a psychopathology built on attachment theory. What guidance does it give for assessing a patient's problems and helping him?

First, we must decide whether the problem presented is one to which attachment theory is applicable, a matter that still requires much exploration. If it seems applicable, we consider what pattern the patient's attachment behaviour typically takes, bearing in mind both what he tells us about himself and the relationships he makes and also how he relates to us as potential helpers. We also explore relevant life events, notably departures, serious illness, or death, and also arrivals, and the degree to which the presenting symptoms can be understood as recent or belated responses to them. During the course of these explorations we may begin to get some inkling of the patterns of interaction that obtain in his present home, which may be either his family of origin or the new family he has helped create, or (perhaps especially in the case of women) both. Any historical material that casts light on how current patterns may have come into being sharpens our perceptions.

A major difficulty in this process of assessment is that the information given may omit vital facts or falsify them. Not only are relatives – parents or spouse – apt to omit, suppress, or falsify but the designated patient may do so as well. This, of course, is no accident. First, it is evident that many parents, who for one reason or another have neglected or rejected a child, have threatened him with abandonment, enacted suicidal attempts, had repeated quarrels between themselves or clung to a child because of their own desire for a care-giving figure, will be loath for the true facts to be known. Inevitably they expect criticism and blame and thus distort the truth, sometimes unwittingly, sometimes deliberately. Similarly, the children of such parents have grown up knowing that the truth must not be divulged and perhaps half-believing also that they themselves are to blame for every trouble, as their parents may always have insisted. A common method of keeping family disturbances a secret is to attribute the symptoms to some other cause; he is afraid of boys at school (not that mother may take her life); she suffers from headaches and indigestion (not that mother threatens to disown her if she leaves home); he was difficult from birth (not that he was unwanted and neglected); she is suffering from an endogenous depression (not that she is belatedly mourning a father lost many years earlier). Time and again what is described as a symptom is found to be a response which, by having become divorced from the situation that elicited it, appears inexplicable. Or else a symptom arises as a result of the patient trying to avoid reacting with genuine feeling to a truly distressing situation. In either case a first and major task is to identify the situation, or situations, to which the patient is either responding or else inhibiting a response.

It is plainly desirable that any clinician undertaking this type of work should have at his disposal an extensive knowledge of deviant patterns of attachment and care-giving behaviour and of the pathogenic family experiences believed commonly to contribute to them; and he should also be familiar with the sorts of information that are frequently omitted, suppressed, or falsified. Given such knowledge it may often be evident that some piece of crucial information is missing and that claims of certain kinds are dubious or clearly false. Above all, a clinician experienced in this work knows when he has yet to discover the facts and is prepared either to wait for the relevant information to emerge or to probe gently into likely areas. Tyros are apt to jump to conclusions and be wrong.

In building up a clinical picture a psychiatrist is wise not to rely on traditional interviewing methods alone but, whenever possible, to engage in one or more family interviews. No other technique is more likely fairly quickly to reveal present patterns in their true light and give clues to how they might have developed. A large number of books on family psychiatry and family therapy are now available. Though they call attention to the immense influence that different patterns of interaction can have on each family member and describe techniques of interviewing and modes of intervention, the concepts they use are not those of attachment theory. For purposes of this exposition therefore they are of limited value.

A great deal of work needs doing before we can be confident which disorders of attachment and care-giving behaviour are treatable by psychotherapy and which not and, if treatable, which of various methods is to be preferred. Much turns on a clinician's experience, capabilities, and facilities. In general, we can follow Malan (1963) in using as a principal criterion whether the designated patient and/or members of his family show a willingness to explore the problem presented along the lines described: whether or not this is so usually emerges during the course of our assessment. Sometimes both designated patient and relatives respond, readily or reluctantly, to the notion that the problem or symptoms complained of seem to make sense in terms of the events and family disturbances they are describing. Not infrequently such ideas are unpalatable to one or more, and on occasion they are rejected as irrelevant and absurd. Depending on these reactions we decide our therapeutic strategy.

There is not space here to consider the uses and limitations of the many possible patterns of therapeutic intervention, either with parents and offspring (of all ages) or with married pairs, that have now become established practice. Joint interviews, individual interviews, alternations of the two, all have their place, and so have prolonged sessions lasting several hours: but we are a long way from knowing which pattern is likely to be best for a given problem. There are, however, certain principles that are relevant to any of these therapeutic procedures. For ease of exposition I take the case of individual therapy; though note that it is possible to rephrase each principle so that it refers to the members of a family instead of to a single person.

As I see it a therapist has a number of interrelated tasks among which are the following:

(a) first, and above all, to provide the patient with a secure base from which he can explore both himself and also his relations with all those with whom he has made, or might make, an affectional bond; and simultaneously to make it clear to him that all the decisions as regards how best to construe a situation and what action is best taken have to be his and that given help we believe him capable of making them;

(b) to join with the patient in such explorations, encouraging him to consider both the situations in which he nowadays tends to find himself with significant persons, and the parts he may play in bringing them about, and also how he responds in feeling, thought, and action when in those situations;

(c) to draw the patient's attention to the ways in which, perhaps unwittingly, he tends to construe the therapist's feelings and behaviour towards him, and to the predictions he (the patient) makes and the actions he takes as a result; and then to invite him to consider whether his modes of construing, predicting, and acting may be partly or wholly inappropriate in the light of what he knows of the therapist;

(d) to help him consider how the situations into which he typically gets himself and his typical reactions to them, including what may be happening between himself and the therapist, may be understood in terms of the real-life experiences he had with attachment figures during his childhood and adolescence (and perhaps may still be having) and of what his responses to them then were (and may still be).

Although the four tasks outlined are conceptually distinct, in practice they have to be pursued simultaneously. For it is one thing for the therapist to do his best to be a reliable, helpful, and continuing figure and another for the patient to construe him and trust him as such. The more unfavourable the patient's experiences with his parents were the less easy is it for him to trust the therapist now and the more readily will he misperceive, misconstrue, and misinterpret what the therapist does and says. Furthermore, the less he can trust the therapist the less will he tell him and the more difficult will it be for both parties to explore the painful or frightening or mysterious events which may have occurred during the patient's earlier years. Finally, the less complete and accurate the picture available of what happened in the past the more difficult the patient's present feelings and behaviour are for both parties to understand, and the more persistent are his misperceptions and misinterpretations likely to be. Thus we find each patient is confined within a more or less closed system and only slowly, often inch by inch, is it possible to help him escape.

Of the four tasks the one that can best wait is consideration of the past since its only relevance lies in the light it throws on the present. The sequence may often be for the therapist and patient, working together, first to recognize that the patient tends habitually to respond to a particular type of interpersonal situation in a certain self-defeating way, next to examine what kinds of feeling and expectation such situations commonly arouse in him, and only after that to consider whether he may have had experiences, recent or long past, which have contributed to his responding with those feelings and expectations in the situations concerned. In this way memories of relevant experiences are evoked, not simply as unhappy occurrences, but in terms of the pervasive influence they are exerting in the present on the patient's feelings, thoughts, and actions.

It is evident that a great many psychotherapists, irrespective of theoretical outlook, habitually address themselves to these tasks so that much of what I am saying will have long been familiar to them. In traditional terminology the tasks are referred to as providing support, interpreting the transference, and constructing or reconstructing past situations. If there are any new points of emphasis in the present formulation they are:

(a) giving a central place, not only in practice but also in theory, to our role of providing a patient with a secure base from which he can explore and then reach his own conclusions and take his own decisions;

(b) abjuring interpretations which postulate various forms of more or less primitive fantasy and concentrating instead on the patient's real-life experiences;

(c) directing attention particularly to the details of how the patient's parents may actually have behaved towards him, not only during his infancy and childhood but during his adolescence and up to the present day as well; and also to how he has commonly responded;

(d) utilizing interruptions in the course of treatment, especially those imposed by the therapist, either routinely as in the case of holidays or exceptionally as in the case of illness, as opportunities first to observe how the patient construes a separation and responds to it, then to help him recognize how he is construing and responding, and finally to examine with him how and why he should have developed so.

An insistence on the principle that a patient's attention should be directed to considering what his real experiences may have been, and how these experiences may still be influencing him, often gives rise to a misunderstanding. Are we doing no more, it may be asked, than encouraging a patient to lay all the blame for his troubles on his parents? and, if so, what good can that do? First, it must be emphasized that, as therapists, it is not our job to determine who is to blame or for what. Instead, our task is to help a patient understand the extent to which he misperceives and misinterprets the doings of those he is fond of or might be fond of in the present day, and how, in consequence, he treats them in ways that have results of a kind he regrets or deplores. Our task, in fact, is to help him review the representational models of attachment figures and of himself that without his realizing it are governing his perceptions, predictions, and actions, and how those models may have developed during his childhood and adolescence and, if he thinks fit, help him to modify them in the light of more recent experience. Second, inasmuch as a patient may be quick to blame, we may be able to point to the emotional difficulties and unhappy experiences his parents may perhaps have had and thus invite his sympathy. Bearing in mind our medical role, we must approach what may be the deeply regrettable behaviour of the patient's parents in as objective a way as we try to approach those of the patient himself. Our role is not to apportion blame but to trace causal chains with a view to breaking them or ameliorating their consequences.

This is a good moment to refer to family therapy, since during the course of family interviews it may be possible to get a much longer perspective on how the current difficulties have come into being. By using such occasions to draw a detailed family tree vital data may be unearthed for the first time, especially when grandparents are included. As a colleague remarks, 'It is amazing to see the effects on a patient of hearing his grandparents talk about their grandparents.'

Although I believe the same principles apply in family therapy as in individual therapy, the differences in application are too many to be dealt with here and deserve a full discussion of their own. One difference may, however, be mentioned. A main aim of family therapy is to enable all members to relate together in such a way that each member can find a secure base in his relationships within the family, as occurs in every healthily functioning family. To this end attention is directed to understanding the ways in which family members may at times succeed in providing each other with a secure base but at other times fail to do so, for example, by misconstruing each other's roles, by developing false expectations of each other, or by redirecting forms of behaviour that would be appropriately directed towards one family member towards another. As a result, during family therapy less time is likely to be given to interpreting the transference than in individual therapy. A main benefit is that, when therapy proves effective, it can often be terminated sooner and with less pain and disturbance than can individual therapy, during the course of which a patient may easily come to regard the therapist as the only secure base he can ever imagine having.

Let us return now to speak again in terms of individual therapy.

I have already emphasized that, in my view, a major therapeutic task is to help a patient discover what the situations are, current or past, to which his symptoms relate, be they either responses to those situations or else the side effects of trying not to respond to them. Yet, since it is the patient who has been exposed to the situations in question, in a sense he is already in possession of all the relevant information. Why then does he need so much help to discover it?

The fact is that much of the most relevant information refers to extremely painful or frightening events that the patient would much prefer to forget. Memories of being held always to be in the wrong, of having to care for a depressed mother instead of being cared for yourself, of the terror and anger you felt when father was violent or mother was uttering threats, of the guilt when you were told your behaviour would make your parent ill, of the grief, despair, and anger you felt after a loss, or of the intensity of your unrequited yearning during a period of enforced separation. No one can look back on such events without feeling renewed anxiety, renewed anger, renewed guilt, or despair. No one, either, cares to believe that it was his very own parents, who at other times may have been kind and helpful, who on occasion behaved in some most distressing way. Nor are parents likely to have encouraged their children to register or to recall such events; all too often indeed they have sought to disconfirm their children's perceptions and have enjoined them to silence. For parents, on their part, to consider in what ways their own behaviour may have contributed and perhaps still be contributing to their child's current problems is equally painful. In all parties, therefore, there are strong pressures towards forgetting and distorting, repressing and falsifying, exonerating one party and blaming another. Thus, we find, defensive processes are as frequently aimed against recognizing or recalling real-life events and the feelings aroused by them as ever they are against becoming aware of unconscious impulse or fantasy. Indeed, it is often only when the detailed course of some disturbed and distressing relationship has been recalled and recounted that the feeling aroused by it and the actions contemplated in reply come to mind. I well remember how a silent inhibited girl in her early twenties given to allegedly unpredictable moods and hysterical outbursts at home responded to my comment 'it sounds to me as though your mother never has really loved you'. (She was the second daughter, to be followed in quick succession by two much-wanted sons.) In a flood of tears she confirmed my view by quoting, verbatim, remarks made by her mother from childhood to the present day, and the despair, jealousy, and rage her mother's treatment roused in her. Discussion of her profound belief that I also found her unlovable and that her relations with me would be as hopeless as they had always been with her mother, which accounted for the sulky silences which had been impeding therapy, followed naturally.

The technique developed for helping bereaved people illustrates well the principles I am describing. In this work, the events in question and the feelings, thoughts, and actions aroused by them are recent and so, compared to childhood events and responses, likely to be more clearly and accurately remembered. Painful feeling, moreover, is often either still present or at least more readily accessible.

Those counselling the bereaved (e.g., Raphael 1975) have found empirically that, if they are to be of help, it is necessary to encourage a client to recall and recount, in great detail, all the events that led up to the loss, the circumstances surrounding it and her experiences since;* for it seems only in this way that a widow, or any other bereaved person, can sort out her hopes, regrets and despairs, her anxiety, anger, and perhaps guilt, and, just as important, review all the actions and reactions that she had it in mind to perform and may still have it in mind to perform, inappropriate or self-defeating though many of them might always have been and would certainly be now. Not only is it desirable for a bereaved person to review everything surrounding the loss but to review also the whole history of the relationship, with all its satisfactions and deficiencies, the things that were done and those that were left undone. For it appears that it is only when she has been able to review and reorganize past experience that it becomes possible for her to consider herself as a widow and her possible futures with their limitations and opportunities, and to make the best of them without subsequent strain or breakdown. The same, of course, applies to widowers and bereaved parents.

Thus far I have not mentioned advice. Experience of bereavement counselling shows that until the bereaved has had time

---

* For demographic reasons the development of techniques of bereavement counselling has been mainly with widows; hence the gender in this paragraph and the next.

to progress some distance in her review of the past and her reorientation towards the future, advice does far more harm than good. Furthermore, what a person needs much more than advice is information. For a widow's situation in life is very different to what it was. Many familiar courses of action are now closed and she may well lack information about those now open to her, with the advantages and disadvantages of each. Providing her with, or guiding her towards, relevant information and helping her review its implications for her future, whilst leaving her to take the decisions, may in due course be very useful. Hamburg has repeatedly emphasized the great importance of a person seeking and utilizing new information as a necessary step in coping with any stressful transition (Hamburg and Adams 1967). Assisting a patient to do so at the right time and in the right way thus constitutes a fifth task for the therapist.

When helping a psychiatric patient the tasks to be undertaken and the techniques for achieving them are, I believe, no different in kind to counselling the bereaved. Such differences as exist are due to the fact that the patient's representational models and the patterns of behaviour based on them have been so long entrenched, that many of the events which led to their development occurred long ago, and that the patient and members of his family may have a deep reluctance to look at things afresh. As a consequence, when helping a psychiatric patient explore his world and himself, a therapist has a complex role to fill.

Thus, he must encourage his patient to explore even when he is resistant to doing so and also help him in the search by drawing attention to features in the story that seem likely to be relevant and away from those that seem irrelevant and distracting. Often he will call a patient's attention to his reluctance even to consider certain possibilities and, perhaps simultaneously, sympathize with the bewilderment, anxiety, and pain that to do so might entail. In all this, it will be noted, I am in agreement with those who believe a therapist's role should be an active one. Yet, to be effective, he must recognize that he cannot go faster than his patient, and that by calling attention to painful topics too insistently he will arouse his patient's fear and earn his anger or deep resentment. Finally, he must never forget that, plausible, even convincing, though his own surmises may seem to him, compared to the patient he is ill-placed to know the facts and that in the long term it is what the patient honestly believes that must be accepted as final.

Here we touch on the immensely important issue of the therapist's own outlook and values in relation to the patient and his or her problems; for whatever the therapist's outlook and attitudes may be are bound to influence the patient's own attitudes, if only through the largely unconscious process of observational learning (identification). In this process the patient's experience of the therapist's behaviour and tone of voice and how he approaches a topic are at least as important as anything he says. Thus, with attachment theory in mind, a therapist will convey, largely by non-verbal means, his respect and sympathy for his patient's desires for love and care from her relatives, her anxiety, anger, and perhaps despair at her wishes having been frustrated and/or denigrated, not only in the past but perhaps also in the present, and the distress and grieving to which perhaps a childhood bereavement may have given rise; and he will indicate his understanding that similar conflicts, expectations, and emotions may be active in the therapeutic relationship as well. As much through non-verbal as through verbal communication also will a therapist convey respect for and encouragement of his patient's desire to explore the world and reach her own decisions in life; whilst at the same time he recognizes that she may have a deep-seated belief, derived from what others have insisted, that she is incapable of doing so. In these everyday exchanges a certain pattern of conducting inter-personal relationships is, unavoidably, demonstrated by the therapist and this cannot but influence in some degree his patient's outlook. For example, in place of what may have been a pattern of fault-finding, punishment, and revenge, or of coercion by induction of guilt, or of evasion and mystification, he introduces a pattern in which an attempt is made to understand another person's viewpoint and to negotiate openly with him. At some points in therapy discussion of these different ways of treating people, and the probable consequences of each, can be useful. During such discussions a therapist is likely both to raise questions and to provide information whilst, once again, leaving the patient to take the decisions.

Clearly, to do this work well requires of the therapist not only a good grasp of principles but also a capacity for empathy and for tolerating intense and painful emotion. Those with a strongly organized tendency towards compulsive self-reliance are illsuited to undertake it and are well advised not to.

In discussing earlier the therapist's four basic tasks it is emphasized that, though conceptually distinct, in practice they have to be pursued simultaneously. How far therapy can and should be taken with any one family or patient is a complex difficult question. The main point perhaps is that a restructuring of a person's representational models and his re-evaluation of some aspects of human relationships, with a corresponding change in his modes of treating people, are likely to be both slow and patchy. In favourable conditions the ground is worked over first from one angle then from another. At best progress follows a spiral. How far a therapist goes and how deeply involved he becomes is a personal matter for both parties. Sometimes one or a few sessions enable a patient or a family to see problems in a new light, or perhaps confirm that a point of view, rejected and ridiculed by others, is indeed plausible and can with advantage be adopted. (See accounts and examples by Caplan 1964; Argles and Mackenzie 1970; Lind 1973; Heard 1974.) A special value of joint family interviews is that they enable each member of a family to discover how each of the others view their family life and to move together in reappraising and changing it. Often, too, they enable all family members to learn, often for the first time, of the unhappy experiences that one or other parent may have had in years past, to the consequences of which current family conflict may quickly be perceived as due. (An excellent example, in which a current marital crisis is traced to the persisting consequences of failed mourning after childhood loss, is described by Paul (1967).) There are many other cases however, especially in patients who have developed a highly organized false self and become compulsively self-reliant or given to the caretaking of others, in which a much longer period of treatment may be necessary before change of any kind is seen.

Nevertheless, however short or long the therapy, evidence is clear that, unless a therapist is prepared to enter into a genuine relationship with a family or individual, no progress can be expected (Malan 1963; Truax and Mitchell 1971). This entails that a therapist should, so far as he can, meet the patient's desire for a secure base, whilst recognizing that his best efforts will fall short of what a patient desires and might well benefit from; that he should enter into the patient's explorations as a companion ready either to take the lead or to be led; and that he should be willing to discuss a patient's perceptions of him and the degree to which they may or may not be appropriate, which is sometimes not easy to determine; and, finally, that he should not pretend otherwise should he become anxious about a patient or irritated by him. This is especially important for those patients whose parents have persistently simulated affection to cover deep seated rejection of them. Guntrip (1975) has well described the therapist's job: 'It is, as I see it, the provision of a reliable and understanding human relationship of a kind that makes contact with the deeply repressed traumatized child in a way that enables [the patient] to become steadily more able to live, in the security of a new real relationship, with the traumatic legacy of the earliest formative years, as it seeps through, or erupts into consciousness.'

When he adopts a stance of this kind a therapist risks certain dangers of which it is as well to be aware. First, a patient's eagerness for a secure base and his tormenting fear he will be rejected may make his claims insistent and difficult to deal with. Second, and far more serious, in exerting these claims a patient may apply to the therapist the very same methods that a parent may have used on him when he was a child. Thus, a man whose mother when he was a boy inverted the relationship by demanding he care for her, and who used either threats or guilt inducing techniques to force him to do so, may during treatment apply these very same techniques to his therapist. Plainly it is of the greatest importance that the therapist should recognize what is happening, trace the origin of the techniques being used and resist them, i.e., set limits. Yet the more subtly guilt-inducing the techniques are and the more eager the therapist is to help, the greater is the danger of his being drawn in. A sequence of this sort, I suspect, accounts for many of the cases described by Balint (1968) as exhibiting 'malignant regression' and classified by others as borderline. The clinical problems to which they can give rise are well illustrated by Main (1957) and also by Cohen et al. (1954). The latter group point to the danger of a therapist not recognizing when a patient's expectations are becoming unrealistic because, when it becomes clear they will not be met, the patient may suddenly feel totally rejected and so despair.

Because attachment theory deals with so many of the same issues as are dealt with by other theories of psychopathology – issues of dependency, object-relations, symbiosis, anxiety, grief, narcissism, trauma, and defensive processes – it is hardly surprising that many of the therapeutic principles to which it leads should be long familiar. Some of the overlaps between ideas I have advanced and those of Balint (1965, 1968), Winnicott (1965) and others have been discussed by Pedder (1976) in connection with the treatment of a depressed patient with a 'false self'. Other overlaps, for example the equivalence of Winnicott's concept of play (Winnicott 1971) and what is here termed exploration, have been noted by Heard (1978). Overlaps with the ideas of therapists who have drawn special attention to the part played in the genesis of episodic depressions and many other neurotic symptoms by the failure to mourn a parent lost during childhood or adolescence (e.g., Deutsch 1937; Fleming and Altschul 1963) or to come to terms with a parent's attempted suicide (Rosen 1955) will be evident. Yet, though these overlaps are real enough, there are significant differences also, both of emphasis and of orientation. They turn partly on how we conceive the place of attachment behaviour in human nature (or, by contrast, what use we make of the concepts of dependency, orality, symbiosis, and regression), and partly on how we believe a person acquires certain disagreeable and self-defeating ways of interacting with those close to him, or misplaced beliefs such as, for example, that he is inherently incapable of doing anything useful or effective.

All those who think in terms of dependency, orality, or symbiosis refer to the expression of attachment desires and behaviour by an adult as being the result of his having regressed to some state believed to be normal during infancy and childhood, often that of a suckling at his mother's breast. This leads therapists to talk to a patient about 'the child part of yourself' or 'your baby need to be loved or fed', and to refer to someone tearful after a bereavement as being in a state of regression. In my view all such statements are mistaken both for theoretical and for practical reasons. As regards theory enough has been said to make it clear that I regard the desire to be loved and cared for as being an integral part of human nature throughout adult life as well as earlier and that the expression of such desires is to be expected in every grown-up, especially in times of sickness or calamity. As regards practice, it seems highly undesirable to refer to a patient's 'baby needs' when we are trying to help him recover his natural desires to be loved and cared for which, because of unhappy experiences earlier in his life, he has endeavoured to disclaim. By construing them as childish and referring to them as such, a patient can easily interpret our remarks as disparaging and reminiscent of a disapproving parent who rejects a child seeking to be comforted and calls him 'silly and babyish'. An alternative way of referring to a patient's desires is to refer to his yearning to be loved and cared for which we all have but which in his case went underground when he was a child (for reasons we may then be able to specify).*

A second area of difference concerns how we suppose a person comes to apply to spouse and children, and sometimes also to therapist, certain disagreeable pressures, for example threats of suicide or subtle modes of inducing guilt. In the past, though the problem has been recognized, no great attention has been given to the possibility that the patient learned how to exert these pressures through having suffered them himself when a child and, consciously or unconsciously, is now copying his parent.

A third area of difference concerns the origin of prolonged despair and helplessness. Traditionally this has been traced, almost solely, to the effects of unconscious guilt. The view I favour, which is in keeping with Seligman's studies of learned helplessness (Seligman 1975) and is also compatible with the traditional view, is that someone who is readily plunged into prolonged moods of hopelessness and helplessness has been exposed repeatedly during infancy and childhood to situations in which his attempts to influence his parents to give him more

* The distinctions I am making are identical to those made by Neki (1976) who contrasts the value set by Indian culture on 'strong interdependent affiliative attachments fostered and carried over into adulthood' with the Western value of 'achievement-oriented independence'. His discussion of how these divergent ideals affect therapy in these respects follows lines closely similar to those sketched here.

time, affection, and understanding have met with nothing but rebuff and punishment.

Finally, we may ask, what evidence is there that therapy conducted according to the principles outlined is effective and, if so, in what types of case? The answer is that there is no direct evidence because no series of patients have been treated along exactly these lines so that no investigation of results has been possible. The most that can be said is that certain indirect evidence is hopeful. It comes from investigations of the efficacy of brief psychotherapy and of bereavement counselling.

For many years Malan (1963, 1973) has been examining the results of brief psychotherapy (defined arbitrarily as no more than forty sessions) and has concluded that a group of patients can be specified who are likely to benefit from a certain type of psychotherapy the features of which can also be specified. The patients likely to benefit are those who, during the first few interviews, show themselves able to face emotional conflict and are willing to explore feelings and to work within a therapeutic relationship. The technique that proved effective was one in which the therapist felt able to understand his patient's problems and to formulate a plan; and in which he attended to the transference relationship and interpreted it boldly, paying especial attention to the patient's anxiety and anger when the therapist set a date for termination.

During the course of a replication study Malan and his colleagues reached the same conclusion. In addition they found evidence that 'an important therapeutic factor is the patient's willingness to involve himself in a way that repeats a childhood relationship' with one or both of his parents and his ability, with the therapist's help, to recognize what is happening (Malan 1973). A further study by the same group, this time of patients who improve after no more than a single interview, presents further evidence in support of that conclusion (Malan et al. 1975).

Although the theory of psychopathology used by Malan and

his colleagues differs in some respects from the one outlined here, there are important similarities. Furthermore, as will be noted, there is considerable similarity between the principles of technique he finds effective and those advocated here.

Evaluation of the efficacy of bereavement counselling for widows thought to have a bad prognosis also points in a hopeful direction. Amongst widows who received the form of counselling described above, significantly more were found, at the end of thirteen months, to have progressed favourably than amongst those in a control group who received no counselling (Raphael and Maddison 1976).

It must, of course, be recognized that to outline principles of therapy is a great deal easier than to apply them in the ever varying conditions of clinical practice. Furthermore, the theory itself is still at an early stage of development and a great deal of work is still to be done. Among priority tasks are to determine both the range of clinical conditions to which the theory is relevant and the particular variants of technique best suited to treat them.

Meanwhile those who adopt attachment theory believe that both its structure and its relation to empirical data are now such that its usefulness can be tested systematically. In the fields of aetiology and psychopathology it can be used to frame specific hypotheses which relate different forms of family experience to different forms of psychiatric disorder and also, it may be, to the neurophysiological changes that accompany them as Hamburg and his colleagues (1974) believe. In the field of psychotherapy it can be used to specify therapeutic technique, to describe therapeutic process and, given the necessary technical developments, to measure change. As research proceeds the theory itself will no doubt be modified and amplified. This gives hope that, in due course, attachment theory may prove useful as one component within that larger corpus of psychiatric science which Henry Maudsley did his utmost to foster.

NOTES

1   Other clinically relevant fields to which attachment theory has been effectively applied are the origins of mother-infant bonding during the neonatal period by Marshall Klaus and John Kennell (1976), disturbances within the marital relationship by Janet Mattinson and Ian Sinclair (1979), and the emotional consequences of marital separation by Robert S. Weiss (1975). Volume 3 of *Attachment and Loss* is due to be published early in 1980.

2   In Chapters 4 and 20 of *Attachment and Loss* Volume 3 I have given a sketch of how defensive processes can be approached in terms of human information processing. See also the monograph by Emanuel Peterfreund (1971).

REFERENCES

Abraham, K. (1924) A Short Study of the Development of the Libido Viewed in the Light of Mental Disorders. In *Selected Papers on Psycho-analysis*. London: Hogarth Press 1927.

Adam, K. S. (1973) Childhood Parental Loss, Suicidal Ideation and Suicidal Behaviour. In E. J. Anthony and C. Koupernik (eds.), *The Child in his Family* Volume 2. New York: John Wiley.

Ahrens, R. (1954) Beitrag zur Entwicklung des Physiognomie – und Mimikerkennes. *Zeitschrift für Experimentelle und Angewandte Psychologie* **11**(3): 412–454.

Ainsworth, M. D. S. (1962) The Effects of Maternal Deprivation: a Review of Findings and Controversy in the Context of Research Strategy. In *WHO Public Health Papers No. 14*. Geneva: World Health Organisation.

—— (1967) *Infancy in Uganda: Infant Care and the Growth of Attachment*. Baltimore: The Johns Hopkins Press.

—— (1969) Object Relations, Dependency and Attachment: a Theoretical Review of the Infant–Mother Relationship. *Child Development* **40**: 969–1027.

—— (1977) Social Development in the First Year of Life: Maternal Influences on Infant–Mother Attachment. In J. M. Tanner (ed.), *Developments in Psychiatric Research*. London: Hodder & Stoughton.

Ainsworth, M. D. S. and Bell, S. M. (1970) Attachment, Exploration and Separation: Illustrated by the Behaviour of One-Year-Olds in a Strange Situation. *Child Development* **41**: 49–67.

Ainsworth, M. D. S., Bell, S. M., and Stayton, D. J. (1971) Individual Differences in Strange-Situation Behaviour of One-Year-Olds. In H. R. Schaffer (ed.), *The Origins of Human Social Relations*. New York: Academic Press.

—— (1974) Infant–Mother Attachment and Social Development: 'Socialization' as a Product of Reciprocal Responsiveness to Signals. In M. P. M. Richards (ed.), *The Integration of a Child into a Social World*. Cambridge: Cambridge University Press.

Ainsworth, M. D. S., Blehar, M. C., Waters, E., and Wall, S. (1978) *Patterns of Attachment: Assessed in the Strange Situation and at Home*. Hillsdale, N.J.: Lawrence Erlbaum.

Ainsworth, M. D. S. and Bowlby, J. (1954) Research Strategy in the Study of Mother–Child Separation. *Courrier de la Centre Internationale de l'Enfance* **4**: 105–131.

Ambrose, J. A. (1963) The Concept of a Critical Period for the Development of Social Responsiveness. In B. M. Foss (ed.), *Determinants of Infant Behaviour* Volume 2. London: Methuen.

Anderson, J. W. (1972) Attachment Behaviour Out of Doors. In N. Blurton Jones (ed.), *Ethological Studies of Human Behaviour*. Cambridge: Cambridge University Press.

Anon (1955) Unhappiness Begins at Home. *Picture Post*: 31st December 1955.

Argles, P. and Mackenzie, M. (1970) Crisis Intervention with a Multi-Problem Family: a Case Study. *Journal of Child Psychology and Psychiatry* **11**: 187–199.

Aubry, J. (1955) *La Carence Des Soins Maternels*. Paris: Presses Universitaires de France.

Balint, M. (1965) *Primary Love and Psychoanalytic Technique*. London: Tavistock Publications.

—— (1968) *The Basic Fault*. London: Tavistock Publications.

Barnes, M. J. (1964) Reactions to the Death of a Mother. *Psychoanalytic Study of the Child* **19**: 334–357.

Bateson, P. P. G. (1966) The Characteristics and Context of Imprinting. *Biological Review* **41**: 177–220.

Baumrind, D. (1967) Child Care Practices Anteceding Three Patterns of Preschool Behaviour. *Genetic Psychology Monographs* **75**: 43–88.

Beach, F. A. and Jaynes, J. (1966) Studies of Maternal Retrieving in Rats.

III Sensory Cues Involved in the Lactating Female's Response to her Young. *Behaviour* **10**: 104–125.

Bischof, M. (1975) A Systems Approach Toward the Functional Connections of Attachment and Fear. *Child Development* **46**: 801–807.

Blurton Jones, N. (ed.) (1972) *Ethological Studies of Child Behaviour.* Cambridge: Cambridge University Press.

Bowlby, J. (1940) The Influence of Early Environment in the Development of Neurosis and Neurotic Character. *International Journal of Psychoanalysis* **21**: 154–178.

—— (1944) Forty-four Juvenile Thieves: Their Characters and Home Life. *International Journal of Psychoanalysis* **25**: 19–52 and 107–127. Reprinted (1946) as monograph. London: Bailliere, Tindall & Cox.

—— (1951) Maternal Care and Mental Health. World Health Organization Monograph Series No. 2. Geneva: World Health Organization. Reprinted (1966) New York: Schocken Books.

—— (1953) Some Pathological Processes Set in Train by Early Mother–Child Separation. *Journal of Mental Science* **99**: 265–272.

—— (1958) The Nature of the Child's Tie to his Mother. *International Journal of Psychoanalysis* **39**: 350–373.

—— (1960a) Separation Anxiety. *International Journal of Psychoanalysis* **41**: 89–113.

—— (1960b) Grief and Mourning in Infancy and Early Childhood. *The Psychoanalytic Study of the Child* **15**: 9–52.

—— (1961a) Separation Anxiety: a Critical Review of the Literature. *Journal of Child Psychology and Psychiatry* **1**: 251–269.

—— (1961b) Processes of Mourning. *International Journal of Psychoanalysis* **42**: 317–340.

—— (1961c) Childhood Mourning and its Implications for Psychiatry. *American Journal of Psychiatry* **118**: 481–498.

—— (1963) Pathological Mourning and Childhood Mourning *Journal of the American Psychoanalytic Association* **11**: 500–541.

—— (1968) Effects on Behaviour of Disruption of an Affectional Bond. In J. M. Thoday and A. S. Parkes (eds.), *Genetic and Environmental Influences on Behaviour.* Edinburgh: Oliver & Boyd.

—— (1969) *Attachment and Loss* Volume 1: *Attachment.* London: Hogarth Press. New York: Basic Books. Harmondsworth: Penguin Books (1971).

—— (1973) *Attachment and Loss* Volume 2: *Separation: Anxiety and Anger.* London: Hogarth Press. New York: Basic Books. Harmondsworth: Penguin Books (1975).

—— (1975) Attachment Theory, Separation Anxiety and Mourning. In S. Arieti (ed.), *American Handbook of Psychiatry* (second edition). New York: Basic Books.

—— (1979) Psychoanalysis as Art and Science. *International Review of Psychoanalysis* **6**: 3–14.

—— (in press) *Attachment and Loss* Volume 3: *Loss*. London: Hogarth Press. New York: Basic Books.

Brackbill, Y. (1956) *Smiling in Infants: Relative Resistance to Extinction as a Function of Reinforcement Schedule*. Stanford University: Ph.D. Thesis.

Brown, F. (1961) Depression and Childhood Bereavement. *Journal of Mental Science* **107**: 754–777.

Brown, F. and Epps, P. (1966) Childhood Bereavement and Subsequent Crime. *British Journal of Psychiatry* **112**: 1043–1048.

Brown, G. W. and Harris, T. (1978) *Social Origins of Depression*. London: Tavistock Publications.

Bruhn, J. G. (1962) Broken Homes Among Attempted Suicides and Psychiatric Outpatients: a Comparative Study. *Journal of Mental Science* **108**: 772–779.

Burlingham, D. and Freud, A. (1942) *Young Children in War-Time London*. London: Allen & Unwin.

—— (1944) *Infants Without Families*. London: Allen & Unwin.

Cairns, R. B. (1966) Attachment Behaviour of Mammals. *Psychological Review* **73**: 409–426.

Caplan, G. (1964) *Principles of Preventive Psychiatry*. New York: Basic Books. London: Tavistock Publications.

Cohen, M. B., Baker, G., Cohen, R. A., Fromm-Reichmann, F., and Weigert, E. (1954) An Intensive Study of Twelve Cases of Manic-Depressive Psychosis. *Psychiatry* **17**: 103–137.

Craft, M., Stephenson, G., and Granger, C. (1964) The Relationship Between Severity of Personality Disorder and Certain Adverse Childhood Influences. *British Journal of Psychiatry* **110**: 392–396.

Darwin, C. (1859) *The Origin of Species by Means of Natural Selection*. London: Murray.

—— (1872) *The Expression of the Emotions in Man and Animals*. London: Murray.

Davis, C. M. (1939) Results of the Self-Selection of Diets by Young Children. *Canadian Medical Association Journal* **41**: 257–261.

Dennehy, C. M. (1966) Childhood Bereavement and Psychiatric Illness. *British Journal of Psychiatry* **110**: 1049–1069.

Dennis, W. (1935) An Experimental Test of Two Theories of Social Smiling in Infants. *Journal of Social Psychology* **6**: 214–223.

Deutsch, H. (1937) Absence of Grief. *Psychoanalytic Quarterly* **6**: 12–22.

Deutsch. J. A. (1953) A New Type of Behaviour Theory. *British Journal of Psychology* **44**: 304–317.

Dollard, J. and Miller, N. E. (1950) *Personality and Psychotherapy*. New York: McGraw-Hill.

Earle, A. M. and Earle, B. V. (1961) Early Maternal Deprivation and Later Psychiatric Illness. *American Journal of Orthopsychiatry* **31**: 181–186.

Engel, G. (1961) Is Grief a Disease? *Psychosomatic Medicine* **23**: 18–22.

Erdelyi, M. H. (1974) A New Look at the New Look: Perceptual Defense and Vigilance. *Psychological Review* **81**: 1–25.

Erikson, E. H. (1950) (revised 1963) *Childhood and Society*. New York: Norton.

Fairbairn, W. R. D. (1952) *Psychoanalytic Studies of the Personality*. London: Tavistock Publications.

Fleming, J. and Altschul, S. (1963) Activation of Mourning and Growth by Psychoanalysis. *International Journal of Psychoanalysis* **44**: 419–431.

Freud, A. (1960) Discussion of 'Grief and Mourning in Infancy and Early Childhood' by John Bowlby. *Psychoanalytic Study of the Child* **15**: 53–62.

Freud, A. and Burlingham, D. (1943) *War and Children*. New York: International Universities Press.

Freud, E. L. (ed.) (1961) *Letters of Sigmund Freud*. London: Hogarth Press.

Freud, S. (1900) *The Interpretation of Dreams* S.E.4.* London: Hogarth Press.

—— (1909) *A Case of Obsessional Neurosis* S.E.10. London: Hogarth Press.

—— (1912) *The Dynamics of the Transference* S.E.12. London: Hogarth Press.

—— (1902–1913) *Totem and Taboo* S.E.13. London: Hogarth Press.

—— (1915) *Instincts and Their Vicissitudes* S.E.14. London: Hogarth Press.

—— (1917) *Mourning and Melancholia* S.E.14. London: Hogarth Press.

—— (1923) *The Ego and the Id* S.E.19. London: Hogarth Press.

—— (1926) *Inhibitions, Symptoms and Anxiety* S.E.20. London: Hogarth Press.

—— (1927) *Fetishism* S.E.21. London: Hogarth Press.

* The abbreviation S.E. in this list of references denotes the Standard Edition of *The Complete Psychological Works of Sigmund Freud*, published in twenty-four volumes by the Hogarth Press, London.

—— (1938) *An Outline of Psychoanalysis* S.E.23. London: Hogarth Press.

—— (1954) *The Origins of Psychoanalysis: Letters to Wilhelm Fliess. Drafts and Notes: 1887–1902.* London: Imago.

Furman, E. (1974) *A Child's Parent Dies: Studies in Childhood Bereavement.* New Haven and London: Yale University Press.

Gero, G. (1936) The Construction of Depression. *International Journal of Psychoanalysis* **17**: 423–461.

Gewirtz, J. L. (1956) A Program of Research on the Dimensions and Antecedents of Emotional Dependence. *Child Development* **27**: 205–221.

Gewirtz, J. L. (ed.) (1972) *Attachment and Dependency.* Washington: V. H. Winston.

Glick, I. O., Weiss, R. S., and Parkes, C. M. (1974) *The First Year of Bereavement.* New York: John Wiley.

Goldfarb, W. (1955) Emotional and Intellectual Consequences of Psychological Deprivation in Infancy: a Revaluation. In P. H. Hoch and J. Zubin (eds.), *Psychopathology of Childhood.* New York: Grune & Stratton.

Greer, S. (1964a) Study of Parental Loss in Neurotics and Psychopaths. *Archives of General Psychiatry* **11**: 177–180.

—— (1964b) The Relationship Between Parental Loss and Attempted Suicide: a Control Study. *British Journal of Psychiatry* **110**: 698–705.

Greer, S. and Gunn, J. C. (1966) Attempted Suicides From Intact and Broken Parental Homes. *British Medical Journal* **2**: 1355–1357.

Greer, S., Gunn, J. C., and Koller, K. M. (1966) Aetiological Factors in Attempted Suicide. *British Medical Journal* **2**: 1352–1355.

Grinker, R. R. Sr. (1962) 'Mentally Healthy' Young Males (Homoclites). *Archives of General Psychiatry* **6**: 405–453.

Guntrip, H. (1975) My Experience of Analysis with Fairbairn and Winnicott. *International Review of Psychoanalysis* **2**: 145–156.

Hamburg, D. A. and Adams, J. E. (1967) A Perspective on Coping Behaviour. *Archives of General Psychiatry* **17**: 277–284.

Hamburg, D.A., Hamburg, B. A., and Barchas, J. D. (1974) Anger and Depression in Perspective of Behavioural Biology. In L. Levi (ed.), *Parameters of Emotion.* New York: Raven Press.

Harlow, H. F. (1958) The Nature of Love. *American Journal of Psychology* **13**: 673–685.

Harlow, H. F. and Harlow, M. R. (1965) The Affectional Systems. In A. M. Schrier, H. F. Harlow, and F. Stollnitz (eds.), *Behaviour of Non-Human Primates* Volume 2. New York and London: Academic Press.

Harlow, H. F. and Zimmerman, R. R. (1959) Affectional Responses in the Infant Monkey. *Science* **130**: 421–432.

Heard, D. H. (1974) Crisis Intervention Guided by Attachment Concepts: a Case Study. *Journal of Child Psychology and Psychiatry* **15**: 111–122.

—— (1978) From Object Relations to Attachment: a Framework for Family Therapy. *British Journal of Medical Psychology* **51**: 67–76.

Heathers, G. (1955) Acquiring Dependence and Independence: a Theoretical Orientation. *Journal of Genetic Psychology* **87**: 277–291.

Heinicke, C. M. (1956) Some Effects of Separating Two-Year-Old Children From Their Parents: a Comparative study. *Human Relations* **9**: 105–176.

Heinicke, C. and Westheimer, I. (1966) *Brief Separations*. New York: International Universities Press. London: Longmans.

Henderson, A. S. (1974) Care-Eliciting Behaviour in Man. *Journal of Nervous and Mental Disease* **159**: 172–181.

Hilgard, J. R. and Newman, M. F. (1959) Anniversaries in Mental Illness. *Psychiatry* **22**: 113–121.

Hilgard, J. R., Newman, M. F., and Fisk, F. (1960) Strength of Adult Ego Following Childhood Bereavement. *American Journal of Orthopsychiatry* **30**: 788–789.

Hill, O. W. and Price, J. S. (1967) Childhood Bereavement and Adult Depression. *British Journal of Psychiatry* **113**: 743–751.

Hinde, R. A. (1954) Changes in Responsiveness to a Constant Stimulus. *Animal Behaviour* **2**: 41–55.

—— (1970) *Animal Behaviour: a Synthesis of Ethology and Comparative Psychology* (second edition). New York: McGraw-Hill.

—— (1974) *Biological Bases of Human Social Behaviour*. New York and London: McGraw-Hill.

Hinde, R. A. and Spencer-Booth, Y. (1967) The Behaviour of Socially Living Rhesus Monkeys in Their First Two and a Half Years. *Animal Behaviour* **15**: 169–196.

—— (1971) Effects of Brief Separation From Mother in Rhesus Monkeys. *Science* **173**: 111–118.

Home Office (1955) *Seventh Report on the Work of the Children's Department*. London: H.M.S.O.

Hunt, J. McV. (1941) The Effects of Infant Feeding Frustration Upon Adult Hoarding in the Albino Rat. *Journal of Abnormal and Social Psychology* **36**: 338–360.

Illingworth, R. S. and Holt, K. S. (1955) Children in Hospital: Some

Observations on Their Reactions with Special Reference to Daily Visiting. *Lancet* ii: 1257–1262.

Jacobson, E. (1943) The Oedipus Conflict in the Development of Depressive Mechanisms. *Psychoanalytic Quarterly* **12**: 541–560.

—— (1946) The Effect of Disappointment on Ego and Superego Formation in Normal and Depressive Development. *Psychoanalytic Review* **33**: 129–147.

—— (1957) Normal and Pathological Moods: Their Nature and Functions. *Psychoanalytic Study of the Child* **12**: 73–113.

Jersild, A. T. (1943) Studies of Children's Fears. In R. G. Barker and H. F. Wright (eds.), *Child Behaviour and Development*. New York and London: McGraw-Hill.

—— (1947) *Child Psychology* (third edition). London: Staples Press.

Jersild, A. T. and Holmes, F. B. (1935) Children's Fears. *Columbia University Child Development Monograph No. 20*.

Kessel, N. (1965) Self-Poisoning. *British Medical Journal* **2**: 1265–1270 and 1336–1340.

Klaus, M. H. and Kennell, J. H. (1976) *Maternal-Infant Bonding*. St. Louis: Mosby.

Klein, M. (1935) A Contribution to the Psychogenesis of Manic-Depressive States. In *Contributions to Psychoanalysis 1921–1945*. London: Hogarth Press (1948)

—— (1940) Mourning and Its Relation to Manic-Depressive States. In *Contributions to Psychoanalysis 1921–1945*. London: Hogarth Press (1948)

—— (1948) *Contributions to Psychoanalysis 1921–1945*. London: Hogarth Press. New York: Hillary.

Korchin, S. J. and Ruff, G. E. (1964) Personality Characteristics of the Mercury Astronauts. In C. H. Grosser, H. Wechsler, and M. Greenblatt (eds.), *The Threat of Impending Disaster: Contributions to the Psychology of Stress*. Cambridge, Mass.: M.I.T. Press.

Lewis, A. (1951) The Twenty-Fifth Maudsley Lecture. Henry Maudsley: His Work and Influence. *Journal of Mental Science* **97**: 259–277.

—— (1967) Problems Presented by the Ambiguous Word 'Anxiety' as Used in Psychopathology. *Israel Annals of Psychiatry and Related Disciplines* **5**: 105–121.

Lind, E. (1973) From False-Self to True-Self Functioning: a Case in Brief Psychotherapy. *British Journal of Medical Psychology* **46**: 381–389.

Lindemann, E. (1944) Symptomatology and Management of Acute Grief. *American Journal of Psychiatry* **101**: 141–148.

Lorenz, K. Z. (1935) Der Kumpan in der Umwelt des Vogels. *Journal of Ornithology, Leipzig* **83** (English translation: In C. Schiller (ed.) (1957), *Instinctive Behaviour*. New York: International Universities Press).

—— (1950) The Comparative Method in Studying Innate Behaviour Patterns. In *Physiological Mechanisms in Animal Behaviour* (No. 17 of Symposia of the Society for Experimental Biology). Cambridge: Cambridge University Press.

—— (1956) Comparative Behaviourology. In J. M. Tanner and B. Inhelder (eds.), *Discussions on Child Development* Volume 1. London: Tavistock Publications.

Maccoby, E. E. and Masters, J. C. (1970) Attachment and Dependency. In P. H. Mussen (ed.), *Carmichael's Manual of Child Psychology* (third edition). New York and London: John Wiley.

Maddison, D. and Walker, W. L. (1967) Factors Affecting the Outcome of Conjugal Bereavement. *British Journal of Psychiatry* **113**: 1057–1067.

Main, T. F. (1957) The Ailment. *British Journal of Medical Psychology* **30**: 129–145.

Malan, D. M. (1963) *A Study of Brief Psychotherapy*. London: Tavistock Publications.

—— (1973) Therapeutic Factors in Analytically-Oriented Brief Psychotherapy. In R. H. Gosling (ed.), *Support, Innovation, and, Autonomy*. London: Tavistock Publications.

Malan, D. M., Heath, E. S., Bacal, H. A., and Balfour, F. H. G. (1975) Psychodynamic Changes in Untreated Neurotic Patients: II. Apparently Genuine Improvements. *Archives of General Psychiatry* **32**: 110–126.

Marris, P. (1958) *Widows and Their Families*. London: Routledge & Kegan Paul.

Mattinson, J. and Sinclair, I. A. C. (1979) *Mate and Stalemate: Working With Marital Problems in a Social Services Department*. Oxford: Blackwell.

Ministry of Education (1955) *Report of the Committee on Maladjusted Children*. London: H.M.S.O.

Moynihan, M. (1953) Some Displacement Activities of the Black-Headed Gull. *Behaviour* **5**: 58–80.

Munro, A. (1966) Parental Deprivation in Depressive Patients. *British Journal of Psychiatry* **112**: 443–448.

Murphey, E. B., Silber, E., Coelho, G. V., Hamburg, D. A., and Greenberg, I. (1963) Developments of Autonomy and Parent–Child Interaction in Late Adolescence. *American Journal of Orthopsychiatry* **33**: 643–652.

Naess, S. (1962) Mother–Child Separation and Delinquency: Further Evidence. *British Journal of Criminology* **2**: 361–374.

Neki, J. S. (1976) An Examination of the Cultural Relativism of Dependence as a Dynamic of Social and Therapeutic Relationships, Parts 1 and 2. *British Journal of Medical Psychology* **49**: 1–22.

Offer, D. (1969) *The Psychological World of the Teenager*. New York: Basic Books.

Padilla, S. G. (1935) Further Studies on the Delayed Pecking of Chicks. *Journal of Comparative Psychology* **20**: 413–443.

Parkes, C. M. (1965) Bereavement and Mental Illness. *British Journal of Medical Psychology* **38**: 1–26.

—— (1969) Separation Anxiety: an Aspect of the Search for a Lost Object. In M. H. Lader (ed.), *Studies of Anxiety* (British Journal of Psychiatry, Special Publication No. 3). London: Royal Medico: Psychological Association and Headley Press.

—— (1971a) Psycho-Social Transitions: a Field of Study. *Social Science and Medicine* **5**: 101–115.

—— (1971b) The First Year of Bereavement: a Longitudinal Study of the Reactions of London Widows to the Death of Their Husbands. *Psychiatry* **33**: 444–467.

—— (1972) *Bereavement: Studies of Grief in Adult Life*. New York: International Universities Press. London: Tavistock Publications.

—— (1973) Factors Determining the Persistence of Phantom Pain in the Amputee. *Journal of Psychosomatic Research* **17**: 97–108.

Paul, N. L. (1967) The Role of Mourning and Empathy in Conjoint Marital Therapy. In G. H. Zuk and I. Boszormenyi-Nagy (eds.), *Family Therapy and Disturbed Families*. Palo Alto, California: Science & Behaviour Books.

Peck, R. F. and Havighurst, R. J. (1960) *The Psychology of Character Development*. New York: John Wiley.

Pedder, J. (1976) Attachment and New Beginning. *International Review of Psychoanalysis* **3**: 491–497.

Peterfreund, E. (1971) *Information, Systems and Psychoanalysis*. New York: International Universities Press.

Piaget, J. (1937) *The Child's Construction of Reality* (English translation by M. Cook). London: Routledge & Kegan Paul (1955).

Pollock, G. H. (1961) Mourning and Adaptation. *International Journal of Psychoanalysis* **42**: 341–361.

Prugh, D., Staub, E. M., Sands, H. H., Kirschbaum, R. M., and Lenihan, E. A. (1953) Study of Emotional Reactions of Children and Families to Hospitalization and Illness. *American Journal of Orthopsychiatry* **23**: 70–106.

Raphael, B. (1975) Management of Pathological Grief. *Australian and New Zealand Journal of Psychiatry* **9**: 173–180.

Raphael, B. and Maddison, D. C. (1976) The Care of Bereaved Adults. In O. Hill (ed.), *Modern Trends in Psychosomatic Medicine*. London: Butterworths.

Robertson, J. (1953a) *Film: A Two-Year-Old Goes to Hospital*. London: Tavistock Child Development Research Unit. New York: New York University Film Library.

—— (1953b) Some Responses of Young Children to Loss of Maternal Care. *Nursing Times* **49**: 382–386.

Robertson, J. and Bowlby, J. (1952) Responses of Young Children to Separation From Their Mothers. *Courrier de la Centre Internationale de l'Enfance* **2**: 131–142.

Robertson, J. and Robertson, J. (1967–72) *Young Children in Brief Separation* (Film series). London: Tavistock Institute of Human Relations.

Rollman-Branch, H. S. (1960) On the Question of Primary Object Need. *Journal of the American Psychoanalytic Association* **8**: 686–702.

Root, N. (1957) A Neurosis in Adolescence. *Psychoanalytic Study of the Child* **12**: 320–334.

Rosen, V. H. (1955) The Reconstruction of a Traumatic Childhood Event in a Case of Derealization. *Journal of the American Psychoanalytic Association* **3**: 211–221. Reprinted in A. C. Cain (ed.) (1972), *Survivors of Suicide*. Springfield, Illinois: Thomas.

Roudinesco, J., Nicolas, J., and David, M. (1952) Responses of Young Children to Separation From Their Mothers. *Courrier de la Centre Internationale de l'Enfance* **2**: 68–78.

Rowell, T. E. and Hinde, R. A. (1963) Responses of Rhesus Monkeys to Mildly Stressful Situations. *Animal Behaviour* **11**: 235–243.

Ruff, G. E. and Korchin, S. J. (1967) Adaptive Stress Behaviour. In M. H. Appley and R. Trumbull (ed.), *Psychological Stress*. New York: Appleton–Century–Crofts.

Sade, D. S. (1965) Some Aspects of Parent-Offspring and Sibling Relations in a Group of Rhesus Monkeys, With a Discussion of Grooming. *American Journal of Anthropology* **23**: 1–18.

Schaffer, H. R. (1958) Objective Observations of Personality Development in Early Infancy. *British Journal of Medical Psychology* **31**: 174–183.

Schaffer, H. R. and Callender, W. M. (1959) Psychological Effects of Hospitalization in Infancy. *Pediatrics* **24**: 528–539.

Schaffer, H. R. and Emerson, P. (1964) The Development of Social

Attachments in Infancy. *Monographs of the Society for Research in Child Development* **29**: 1–77.

Sears, R. R., Maccoby, E. E., and Levin, H. (1957) *Patterns of Child Rearing*. Evanston, Ill.: Row, Peterson.

Seligman, M. E. P. (1975) *Helplessness: on Depression, Development and Death*. San Francisco: Freeman.

Sluckin, W. (1964) *Imprinting and Early Learning*. London: Methuen.

Spencer-Booth, Y. and Hinde, R. A. (1966) The Effects of Separating Rhesus Monkey Infants From Their Mothers for Six Days. *Journal of Child Psychology and Psychiatry* **7**: 179–198.

Spitz, R. A. (1946) Anaclitic Depression. *Psychoanalytic Study of the Child* **2**: 313–342.

Spitz, R. A. and Wolf, K. M. (1946) The Smiling Response: a Contribution to the Ontogenesis of Social Relations. *Genetic Psychology Monographs* **34**: 57–125.

Stengel, E. (1939) Studies on the Psychopathology of Compulsive Wandering. *British Journal of Medical Psychology* **18**: 250–254.

—— (1941) On the Aetiology of the Fugue States. *Journal of Mental Science* **87**: 572–599.

—— (1943) Further Studies on Pathological Wandering. *Journal of Mental Science* **89**: 224–241.

Stern, D. N. (1977) The First Relationship: Infant and Mother. London: Fontana/Open Books.

Stewart, A. H. *et al.* (1954) Excessive Infant Crying (Colic) in Relation to Parent Behaviour. *American Journal of Psychiatry* **110**: 687–694.

Strachey, A. (1941) A Note on the Use of the Word 'Internal'. *International Journal of Psychoanalysis* **22**: 37–43.

Tanner, J. M. and Inhelder, B. (eds.) (1956) *Discussions on Child Development* Volume 1. (Proceedings of the First Meeting of the World Health Organization Study Group on the Psychobiological Development of the Child). London: Tavistock Publications.

Thorpe, W. H. (1956) *Learning and Instinct in Animals*. London: Methuen.

Tinbergen, N. (1955) Psychology and Ethology as Supplementary Parts of a Science of Behaviour. In B. Schaffner (ed.), *Group Processes I*. New York: Josiah Macy Junior Foundation.

Truax, C. B. and Mitchell, K. M. (1971) Research on Certain Therapist Interpersonal Skills in Relation to Process and Outcome. In A. E. Bergin and S. L. Garfield (eds.), *Handbook of Psychotherapy and Behaviour Change*. New York: John Wiley.

Ucko, L. E. (1965) A Comparative Study of Asphyxiated and Non-

Asphyxiated Boys From Birth to Five Years. *Developmental Medicine and Child Neurology* **7**: 643–657.

Weidmann, U. (1956) Some Experiments on the Following and the Flocking Reaction of Mallard Ducklings. *Animal Behaviour* **4**: 78–79.

Weiss, R. S. (1975) *Marital Separation*. New York: Basic Books.

Wenner, N. K. (1966) Dependency Patterns in Pregnancy. In J. H. Masserman (ed.), *Sexuality of Women*. New York: Grune & Stratton.

Winnicott, D. W. (1965) *The Maturational Processes and the Facilitating Enivironment*. London: Hogarth Press.

—— (1971) *Playing and Reality*. London: Tavistock Publications.

Wolfenstein, M. (1966) How is Mourning Possible? *The Psychoanalytic Study of the Child* **21**: 93–123.

Yerkes, R. M. (1943) *Chimpanzees: a Laboratory Colony*. New Haven: Yale University Press.

INDEX